Intravascular Infusion Systems

Intravascular Infusion Systems

PRINCIPLES AND PRACTICE

Robert K. Ausman, MD

Medical College of Wisconsin and
Good Samaritan Medical Center, Milwaukee, Wisconsin, USA

Published, in association with
Hastings Hilton Publishers Limited,
by

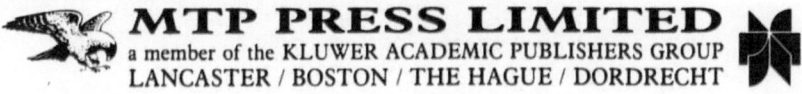

MTP PRESS LIMITED
a member of the KLUWER ACADEMIC PUBLISHERS GROUP
LANCASTER / BOSTON / THE HAGUE / DORDRECHT

MTP PRESS – 10507 – File 150 – T5

Published, in association with Hastings Hilton Publishers, by
MTP Press
A division of Kluwer Boston Inc
190 Old Derby Street
Hingham, MA 02043, USA

Softcover reprint of the hardcover 1st edition 1984

ISBN-13:978-94-011-6343-9   e-ISBN-13: 978-94-011-6341-5
DOI: 10.1007/978-94-011-6341-5

Contents

Contents

Preface

This book has been written for use by health professionals, typically physicians, nurses, and pharmacists, who have a constant relationship with intravascular infusions. It is intended to provide information where appropriate and guidance when possible for the safe and effective use of parenteral fluids.

For several years medical practitioners viewed 'i.v. fluids' rather casually. In as much as the solutions themselves seemed innocuous, these medications did not enjoy the respect given to more potent pharmaceuticals. Intravenous fluid systems were commodities; purchase and use decisions for whole hospitals were placed in the domain of business office personnel. Any tendency toward cessation of 'in hospital manufacture' of solutions was driven by the adverse economics of costly equipment replacement rather than a desire to improve the quality of the product being administered to the patient.

An event in 1971 which changed this environment involved an epidemic of patient infections which were related to a specific solution system. Almost immediately there was an enhanced involvement of health care people who assumed responsibility for i.v. fluids and their use. This intensity of interest has not diminished.

A few years ago publication of this book would not have been possible because there was no audience for it. No one was interested. Now there are many people who want to know and want to become involved. It is my hope those who read this book will not be disappointed.

A special note of my gratitude is due to some colleagues and assistants who helped make this book a reality. Dr Gil Hardy joined me in a several day search through the library at Oxford University for the writings of Sir Christopher Wren. Dr Roy Sanford provided insight into the statistical basis for admixture quality control. Mary Beth Verhetsel was helpful with the chapter on blood administration, and Claudia Teich described the simplified technique for central venous catheter management from the nurse's standpoint. Initially, Mrs Arlene Hoffer and in substantial measure Mrs Sherle Strom prepared several successive drafts of the manuscript. Nearly all of the illustrations were done by Mr Wayne Kos. To these people and others too numerous to mention I am indebted for their support.

Robert K. Ausman, MD
Long Grove, Illinois
January, 1984

7

1
History of I.V. Infusions

In the riches which come to all who undertake the care of their fellow man is the heritage which forms the basis of medical care today. Each branch of the medical profession can boast of heroes and heroines who made an indelible imprint by the enunciation of a new principle or the pronouncement of a discovery having unique and signal character. Names such as Hippocrates, Semmelweis, Osler, and Curie recall the glory of the past; a recounting of their achievements should kindle a special enthusiasm among those who come as neophytes to the profession.

The history of intravascular fluid systems cannot be told in exciting and romantic terms, for it is a tale not so much of individuals as of technical development. Certainly some giant steps were made, and for these there are identifiable persons to recognize. In retrospect it seems that little things, cumulative over time and interspersed generously among a few great discoveries, have developed into methodologies of the current era.

These small observations and ideas, each an improvement, were made by talented people who sought to improve methods of health care. For the most part the discoverers and innovators are not remembered; only the results of their efforts live on.

Here are some vignettes which are interesting from several viewpoints. Often they show that the apparatus of the first physicians interested in intravascular infusion was not remarkably different from what is in use today. They reveal capable thinking by scientists who were wise enough to make observations and proceed with actions designed to correct the abnormalities they saw.

Early history does not record any routine method of access to the circulatory system. The anatomy of the vascular system was described

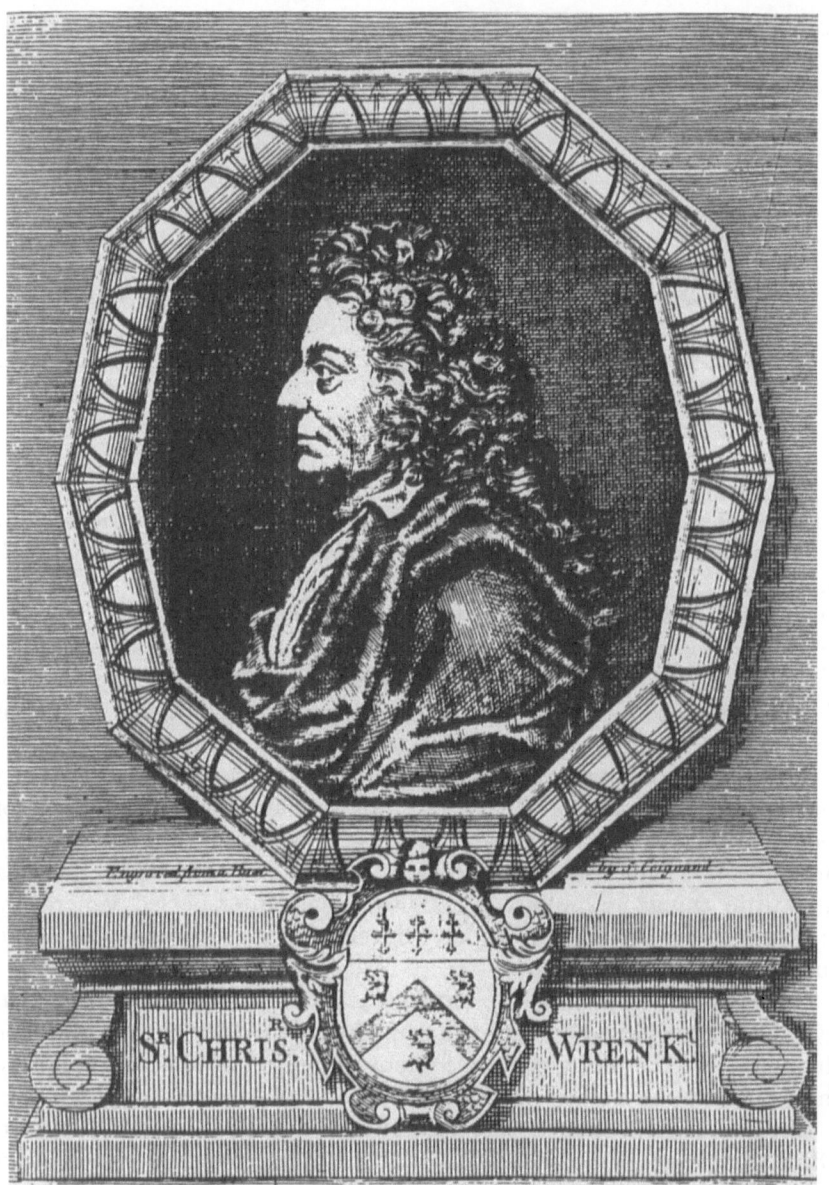

Figure 1.1 Christopher Wren

by Harvey in 1628*. It was Christopher Wren† who established that an avenue to the entire body might be obtained when he cannulated the forearm vein of a dog with a goose quill for the purpose of injecting wine, ale, opium, scammony and other substances. He presented his work initially to his colleagues at Oxford University and later to members of the Royal Society in London. Of his experiments Wren wrote (1656)

'The most considerable experiment I have made of late is this. I injected wine and ale into the mass of blood in a living dog, by a vein, in good quantities, till I made him extremely drunk, but soon after he pissed it out. With two ounces of *Crocus Metallorum* thus injected, the dog immediately fell to vomiting, and so vomited until he died. It will be too long to tell you the effects of Opium, Scammony, and other things which I have tried this way. I am in further pursuit of the experiment which I take to be of great concernment and what will give great Light to the Theory and Practice of Physick'.

Later (*Lancet*, 22, II, 274-281, 1832) Dr Thomas Latta of Leith, Scotland described his 'new' treatment for cholera which was spreading in epidemic form through the country, having been imported from Russia in 1829. His insight into the risks of failure which would doom any new technology teach a valuable lesson.

'I have already given an instance where deficiency in quantity was the cause of failure which I will now contrast with one in which it was used freely. A female, aged 50, very destitute, but previously in good health was on the 13th at four a.m. seized with cholera in its most violent form, and by half past nine was reduced to a most hopeless state. The pulse was quite gone, even in the axilla, and strength so much exhausted that I had resolved not to try the effects of the injection, conceiving the poor woman's case to be hopeless, and that the failure of the experiment might afford the prejudiced and illiberal an opportunity to stigmatise the practice; however, I at length thought I would give her a chance, and in the presence of Dr. Lewins and Craige and Messrs. Sibson and Paterson, I injected one hundred twenty ounces, when like the effects of magic, instead of the pallid aspect of one whom death had sealed as his own, the vital tide was restored and life and vivacity returned'.

The year 1898 produced a profusion of papers on the general subject of infusing saline solution. No less than ten authors reported on various theories, techniques, and experiences. Among them was Thomas Reilly, M.D. (*Medical Record*, 54, 685, 1898).

'The apparatus commonly employed in the hospitals of New York for this purpose (intravenous infusion) consists of a glass funnel connected by a piece of rubber tubing, three feet or more in length, to a cannula, about four inches

---

* *De motre cordis*, W. Harvey 1628.

† Wren is better known for his excellence in architecture. He designed St Paul's Cathedral in London, built among the ashes of its predecessor structure following the great fire which leveled much of that city in 1666. Although his early activities were in medicine, he excelled during his life in astronomy, meteorology and mathematics. He died in 1723 at the age of 91.

An Account of the Rife and Attempts of a Way to convey Liquors immediately into the Mafs of Blood.

Philofophical Tranfactions, No. 7. p. 128. 1665. WHereas there have lately appear'd in publick fome *Books*, printed beyond the Seas, treating of the Way of *injecting Liquors into Veins*; in which Books the *Original* of that *Invention*, feems to be afcrib'd to others, befides him, to whom it really belongs; it will furely not be thought amifs if fomething be faid, whereby the true *Inventor's* Right may beyond Exception be afferted and preferv'd; to which End, there will need no more, than barely to reprefent the *Time* when, and the *Place* where, and among *whom* it was firft ftarted, and put to trial. To join all thefe Circumftances together, 'tis notorious, that at leaft fix Years (a good while before it was heard off, that any one did pretend to have fo much as thought of it) the learned and ingenious Doctor *Chriftopher Wren* did propofe in the *Univerfity* of *Oxford*, (where he now is the worthy *Savilian Profeffor* of *Aftronomy*, and where very many curious Perfons are ready to atteft this Relation) to that noble Benefactor to experimental Philofophy, Mr. *Robert Boyle*, Dr. *Wilkins*, and other deferving Perfons, that he thought, he could eafily contrive a Way, to convey any liquid Thing immediately into the Mafs of Blood, *videl.* by making Ligatures on the Veins, and then opening them on the Side of the Ligature towards the Heart, and by putting into them flender Syringes, or Quills, faften'd to Bladders (in the Manner of Clyfter Pipes) containing the Matter to be injected; performing that Operation upon pretty big and lean Dogs, that the Veffels might be large enough, and eafily acceffible.

This Propofition being made, Mr. *Boyle* foon gave Order for an *Apparatus*, to put it to *Experiment*; wherein at feveral Times, upon feveral *Dogs*, *Opium*, and the Infufion of *Crocus Metallorum* were injected into that Part of the hind Legs of thofe Animals, whence the larger Veffels, that carry the Blood, are moft eafy to be taken hold of; whereof the Succefs was, that the *Opium* being foon circulated into the Brain, did within a fhort Time ftupify, tho' not kill the Dog; but a large Dofe of the *Crocus Metallorum*, made another Dog vomit up Life and all: all which is more amply and circumftantially deliver'd by Mr. *Boyle*, in his excellent Book of the *Ufefulnefs* of *experimental Philofophy*, Part 2. Poftfcript to Effay 2. Where 'tis alfo mention'd, that the Fame of this *Invention*, and of the fucceeding Trials being fpread, and particularly coming to the Knowledge of a foreign Ambaffador, that was curious, and then refided in *London*, it was by him tried with fome *Crocus Metallorum*, upon a Malefactor, that was an inferiour Servant of his; with this Succefs, that the Fellow, as foon as ever the In-

Figure 1.2 A description of the Wren experiments

long by one eighth of an inch in diameter curved for about an inch at its point to facilitate introduction into the vein, and is generally provided with a stopcock'.

Dr Reilly also cast some light on the risks of air infusion (a subject which continues to be poorly understood).

'Contrary to the general opinion there is very little danger to be feared from the introduction of small quantities of air into the circulation ... In one instance Hare injected 40 cubic centimeters of air into the vein of a dog without any evident effect on blood pressure'.

A major continuing problem associated with intravenous fluid administration was pyrogenicity, the occurrence of fever in patients receiving solution by vein. It was the goal of pioneers in the commercial manufacture of parenteral fluids to rid infusions of this adverse reaction by preparing contamination free products which would be both safe and effective for patients compared to materials made in the hospital central supply area. Since 1931 terminally sterilized, pyrogen free, pharmaceutically elegant solution has been available, first in glass bottles and more recently in plastic, flexible, non-air dependent containers.

Now it is possible to access the vascular system and, in the words of Thomas Latta, 'to throw the fluid immediately into the circulation'.

2
Infusion System Designs

This chapter contains a description of the basic container design for each of three fluid infusion systems in general use today. There are at least two reasons why it is important to know how these systems work. When the design theory is understood, it is possible to devise proper methods for use, methods that emphasize system advantages and minimize system risks. When a malfunction occurs, it is very helpful to understand system design features in order to recognize and correct the difficulty quickly.

GLASS CONTAINERS

There are two types of containers, glass and plastic. (In some countries glass containers no longer are available.) Glass is a material with a long and honored history. It was selected originally because it is essentially inert. It can be made in convenient configurations with sufficient wall thickness to withstand minor trauma and internal pressures that develop during sterilization. There are three types of glass, 'imaginatively' designated I, II and III.

Glass	Description	Typical use
I	borosilicate	alkaline solutions
II	dealkalized soda lime	acidic, neutral solutions
III	soda lime	usually not used for parenteral solutions

Source USP XX p. 949

Type II is employed most frequently in commercial manufacture. Special fluids such as bicarbonate solutions require Type I glass to avoid a reaction between .the liquid and the container wall surface with a resultant change in solution pH and particle shedding. This glass is expensive and is an unnecessary cost for most popular solution formulations. Nearly no Type III glass is used now because it is very soft, serves poorly for stability purposes, and causes changes in solution pH over time. Hospital manufacturing facilities sometimes use Type III glass where low price supervenes the appreciation of its inadequacy.

An attractive feature of glass is its clarity before and during use. It can be inspected relatively easily for cleanliness, and the fluid content of the container can be seen well through it.

There are several disadvantages of glass containers but among the most prominent are (1) integrity faults which are easy to precipitate and difficult to find, (2) poor breaking strength, (3) rigidity, and (4) disposability which is complicated and cumbersome. Any recent hospital patient will testify to the noise attendant upon the use of glass containers, seemingly a minor problem except when a person is bed or room confined. This noise is annoying to patients, especially when their rooms are near the nursing station headquarters which is the usual location for the glass disposal site.

Because glass is rigid, air must be admitted to the container if fluid is to evacuate in a streamlined, uninterrupted, controllable flow. The air inflow must occur over a route separate from the fluid outflow path to prevent gurgling and air entrainment in the discharged fluid. There are two common designs to admit air. These competitive methodologies share approximately equal popularity worldwide. They are both *open* systems.

Separate Airway Design

One is a design in which a plastic air tube ('straw') is attached to the undersurface of the bottle stopper and extends nearly the entire inside length of the container. (Figure 2.1). To be efficient it must reach above the surface of the fluid when the bottle is full and inverted. As the solution departs the container through the administration set, air comes in the 'straw' without bubbling through the solution. The source of air is the environment, and the theoretical risk of contamination would appear to be great since there is no attempt made to filter out dust and microbes. Several studies have shown the real incidence of dangerous bacterial proliferation is remarkably small, probably because most solutions do not support growth of bacteria commonly found in the environment and/ or because the particles in admitted air encounter the barrier of surface tension which prevents them from mixing into the liquid. This fact establishes the foundation for two important dictates in using a container with a separate airway:

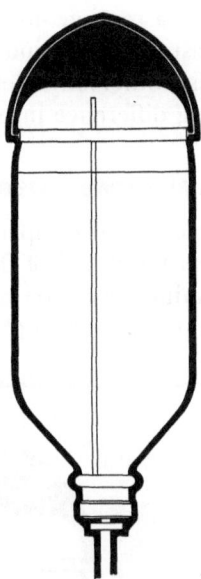

Figure 2.1 Glass container with separate airway

(1) Avoid the temptation to shake the container after it has been hanging in the patient care area and some of the fluid has been discharged. Any particles or organisms which are trapped relatively harmlessly on the surface may be mixed into the solution and infused into the patient.

(2) Allow about 50 ml of fluid to remain in the bottle at the time it is being discontinued or supplanted by a full unit. This last 50 ml will contain most of the particles from the outside air; they could be carried into the patient. The fluid is not 'good to the last drop'.

A difficulty which sometimes becomes extremely aggravating is fluid dripping from the air tube hole in the stopper when the bottle is inverted immediately preceding initiation of fluid flow through the administration set. In times past (uncommonly now because glass systems are less prevalent) it was typical to see nurses with yellow stains on their white uniforms where these drops had fallen (when the solution contained a vitamin additive). This sign identified an individual who had no benefit from in-service education, for the problem can be avoided quite easily. The drops of solution represent a discharge from the air tube of liquid which accumulates while the container is in the upright position. The drops remain there unless a small negative pressure is created as the bottle is turned over. By squeezing and releasing the drip chamber of the

17

attached administration set in a motion simultaneous with inversion of the bottle, this negative pressure can be induced. No dripping ensues, and the system is free of this bothersome deficiency. A small lesson in understanding can make a big difference in performance.

Integral Airway Design

The second kind of glass system is also 'open' in that it requires air to replace the fluid being administered. All of the air bubbles through the solution. Air enters the container via a path in the administration set (Figure 2.2) rather than through a port in a rubber stopper. The entry

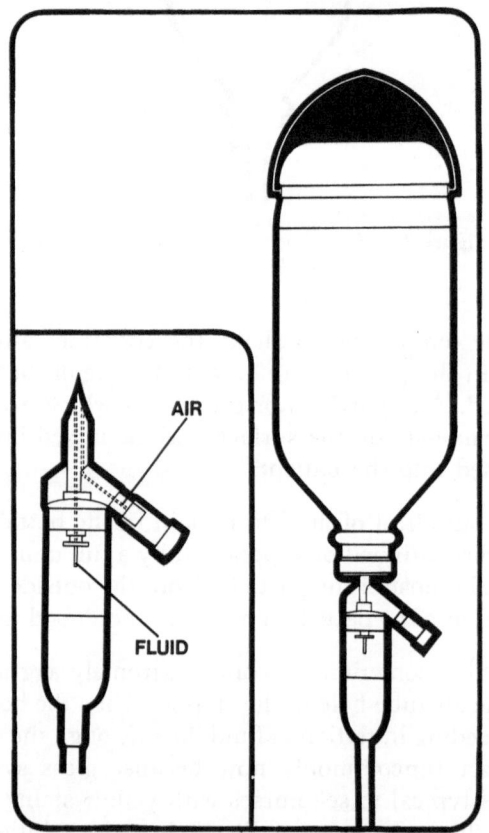

Figure 2.2 Glass container with attached set having an integral airway

site in the set is covered by a filter which provides the proponents of this system a major point of alleged differentiation with the air tube ('straw') design. It is their claim that air entering the solution is sterile because it is filtered, and thus the system is deserving of the descriptive adjective

18

'closed' since it is closed to micro-organisms. Actually this fine point is only hypothetical as it assumes an intact filter. However, the filter cap is removable. The user is encouraged to make any additives necessary during administration of the fluid by removing the filter cap and placing the syringe male end into the air path, then replacing the cap after injecting the syringe contents. If organisms are deposited in the airway during this activity, they are carried into the solution and mixed in it, not layered on top.

Another problem occurs when the filter becomes wet and passes air poorly. When the air filter is clogged or otherwise malfunctioning, only the strongest willed nurse can resist the temptation to remove the cap; when it is removed, unfiltered air *bubbles through* the solution, becomes thoroughly mixed with it, and undoubtedly facilitates the entry of airborne bacteria into the patient's bloodstream. Years ago the airway filter material was cotton; now it is usually cellulose with a more certain and consistent pore size.

In working out new designs, engineers have employed hydrophobic (hates water) filter pads, a seemingly reasonable selection, but filter technology has reached the point of a trade off. Increasing hydrophobia and smaller pore size, two desirable characteristics, can be installed only at the expense of reduced air flow which impedes the exit rate of the infusion fluid. No perfect compromise has been reached.

The set with the airway described above is advertised as self priming, and indeed it is.

CLOSURES FOR GLASS CONTAINERS

For all present types of rigid (glass) containers a standard mix of materials, glass, metal and rubber, comprise the closure system. This arrangement is disadvantageous because of (1) incompatibilities with fluid and additives, and (2) distortion during heat sterilization. The presence in glass containers of discs and stoppers made from a complex milieux of materials can confound any projection of the stability of fluid in the container. When there are several materials, each with a subset of constituents, one or more can participate in a reaction which may end in product deterioration.

Heating to the intense time/temperature levels required to obtain an adequate assurance of sterility results in expansion of metal, rubber and glass which make up the typical rigid container closure. These elements change dimensions at varied rates and in different magnitudes. Measurement tolerances which are critical to the successful function of the closure may be exceeded. Commonly, openings between the exterior environment and interior of the container occur at the peak of heating and early in the cooling phase. This fault has been assigned as the cause for at least one major incident of endogenously (manufacturing source) contaminated fluid in the United States.

PLASTIC CONTAINERS

In 1971 the first extensive commercial marketing of large volume parenteral fluids in a plastic container took place. Originally greeted with some skepticism and reluctance, this configuration captured attention rapidly and now comprises as much as 90–95% of solutions sold and used in many countries. People saw the system as new, but they were unfamiliar with its earlier use by the military during the Vietnam conflict where essentially a total absence of fragility and the ease with which a safe pressure infusion could be performed made it superior to glass. Additional relevant history relates to the plastic blood container which has achieved nearly 100% acceptance in medically advanced countries of the world since its introduction in 1950. Several of the same persons involved in the development of the blood container imparted their technology and expertise to the plastic fluid container.

The principle of operation for the plastic fluid container provides that it is collapsible and requires no admission of air to permit the simultaneous outflow of fluid. Therefore, the flexible plastic container is the only truly *closed* system available. Outside atmospheric pressure pushes evenly (Figure 2.3) on all sides of the container which fall together

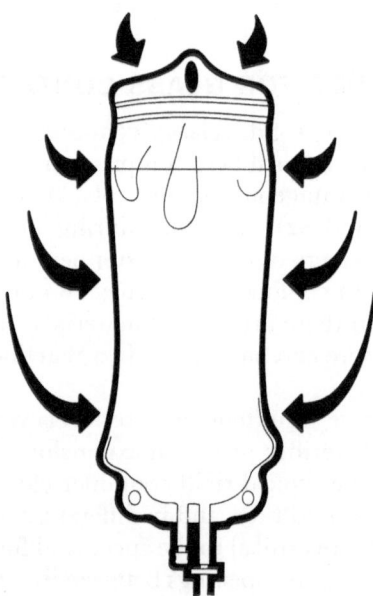

Figure 2.3 Plastic flexible non air dependent container. The arrows indicate the container collapses without admission of air

20

as the fluid drains by gravity. In normal use the plastic container content exits as the result of the force of gravity. Atmospheric pressure does not push the liquid out.

A special feature of the flexible plastic container which contributes to the 'closed' system is the presence of a membrane (Figure 2.4) in each of

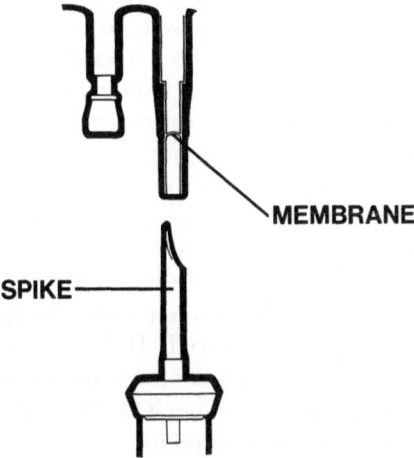

Figure 2.4

the ports which provide access to the container interior. The diameter of the tube where the membrane is located is of a size which tightly surrounds the spike of an administration set as it is inserted. The membrane is placed at a sufficient distance from the tube outlet so that no penetration occurs until the outside environment is sealed off.

The combination of non air dependence and the membrane concept results in no admission of air in the preparation of the infusion and while the solution is being administered. Some individuals have commented that such a design may not be significant in preventing nosocomial (pertaining to a hospital, hospital source) infection arising from contaminated solutions. They support their position by pointing to the lack of evidence for any patient injury (septicemia) ensuing from the admission of air to air dependent containers. They remind us that nearly all environmental micro-organisms are not viable after exposure to the parenteral solutions in common use.

I believe this position is rather tenuous and does not contemplate treatments to which patients are being subjected today. Therapy induced immunosuppression is related to long term treatment of certain conditions. Also, it is known that several disease states are accompanied by relative immunodepression. These patients may be unable to manage the intrusion of viable bacteria as well as persons enjoying relatively good health or an acute, limited illness. Since it has been shown at least

10% of air dependent containers are contaminated during preparation for infusion, the failure to note a significant rate of infection associated with fluid infusion probably is attributable to normal host defense mechanisms. In the immunologically insufficient patient, the defense mechanisms can be malfunctional or absent.

With regard to the hostile environment bacteria encounter when they float on or in solution, it seems hardly wise to plan for their death in this fashion. 'The report of my death is much exaggerated' (Mark Twain, 1897) is a quotation that comes immediately to mind.

The simple fact is that no air enters the closed flexible plastic container, either during preparation or throughout use. There is no risk of fluid contamination or patient injury from this source. Anything different has some probability of contamination, even if it is small. Why accept less than absolute certainty?

There are several unique features of the flexible plastic container. The entire structure which comes in contact with the fluid, including the closure, is made of the same material. It is all polyvinyl chloride or other suitable material; there is no combination of metal, several types of rubber and glass as in rigid systems. Therefore, the study of stability and compatibility with additives is relatively simple, and results often can be extrapolated from basic experiments.

An obvious advantage of the plastic container is that it does not break under normal conditions of use. Drops from a working surface to the floor or from an i.v. pole to the bed where a patient is reclining typically do not result in the fracture of the container or injury to the patient. These accidents are unusual, but they are mentioned by nursing personnel as the primary reason for their preference of the flexible over the rigid container. An added factor is the difference experienced in transporting patients along crowded hallways and on elevators. Clanging bottles have been an ever present hazard nearly everyone remembers. The plastic container has done away with this problem.

In a related design feature the plastic container is fitted with a hanger mechanism which is an inherent part of its structure. The classic metal band and bale (hanger wire) is a thing of the past for plastic units, a happy evolution for pharmacists and nurses who have been cut by sharp metal edges or have seen the metal ring slip from its track and the bottle crash to the floor. Likewise, the basket for the glass container, popular in the United Kingdom, is not necessary when plastic containers are used.

When faced with a need to infuse container contents rapidly, such as Ringer's lactate solution being administered to a patient in shock, the flexible container is supreme. It can be grasped easily and squeezed constantly with nearly no fear of an air embolism. If a semi-automatic mode is desired, the fluid container can be placed in a simple overwrap

22

which has a pneumatic bladder that is inflated to press against the fluid on one side. The amount of air placed in a flexible container during its manufacture or admixture procedures should be monitored carefully so it is always less than the total space remaining within a container squeezed to its limit plus the administration set tubing volume. A greater amount invites the possibility of air embolism. Manufacturers should be asked to certify their design and production techniques for this parameter.

Polyvinyl chloride is the material from which most commercial flexible plastic intravenous solution containers are made. It is the same plastic which has been used in the fabrication of blood containers for many years. A few toxicologists and physicians have challenged the safety of polyvinyl chloride because of the plasticizer component, di-ethyl-hexyl-phthalate (DEHP). In disconnected and questionably relevant experiments, some authors have claimed to show a deleterious effect of DEHP on cells in tissue culture and in some animal systems. A seemingly worrisome carcinogenesis study has been reported within the US government and created much stir in the regulatory agencies charged with protecting public health. As with many similar experiments the dosage of DEHP in these studies had no relation to the real world. (Some manufacturers are offering containers of an alternate material with no DEHP for customers who prefer to avoid the plasticizer; see following description.) One paper has undertaken to establish a connection between pseudomembranous enterocolitis of the newborn and polyvinyl chloride umbilical vein catheters. These assaults have caused several excellent toxicology laboratories to study DEHP rather intensively. The uniform conclusion has been that no adverse effect can be detected. In addition, it has been shown in adult and fetal mice that DEHP is excreted in a rapid and consistent manner both through the kidney and gastrointestinal tract. Tissue distribution studies for several autopsy specimens taken from humans with known different exposures to transfusions of blood showed no difference among the many patients analyzed.

The final and most persuasive evidence in this over dramatized issue relates to the physical/chemical nature of DEHP. Its solubility in water is very low (several faulty experiments have been performed and reported by authors who failed to appreciate this fact). Leaching from the plastic into a solution which is nearly all water is very unlikely. Not only is DEHP not toxic for man, it is not likely to be present in important quantities in solution. This whole description is hardly one of a true and present danger.

Some efforts have been made to utilize a different plastic that contains no leachable materials, expecting the allegedly more inert character will make a safer product. Usually these materials are more rigid than polyvinyl chloride. (One type of molded container does not collapse easily and completely.) The result may be a failure to infuse the entire container contents near the end of the infusion. An easy answer to the problem adopted by one manufacturer has been to increase the container air volume, sometimes to more than 100 ml. This approach is dangerous because the system is closed. Any increase of external pressure on the container when it is empty or nearly so, such as an inadvertent squeeze while changing units, can result in an immediate and sizeable injection of air under positive pressure, an air embolism. There is no justification for accepting such a danger in an intravenous infusion system. The claimed absence of leachables does not create a suitable risk/benefit equation. These units should meet the same performance standards for safety as the polyvinyl chloride container.

There have been some nonpolyvinyl chloride flexible containers tested which appear to meet the requirements of full emptying, small air volume and compatibility with solution. In time they may find a commercial acceptance. Beware the rush to something untested from an article with many miles of experience. The adage about jumping from the frying pan into the fire is worth remembering.

ADMINISTRATION SETS

To deliver fluid from any of the above containers to the patient, an administration set is necessary. Administration sets are the object of much imagination and innovation in an attempt by manufacturers and users to accommodate fluid orders with complicated volumes and sequences, mitigate perceived problems and meet personal preferences. The multitude of designs and configurations makes a description of anything but the basic equipment a very difficult matter. Suffice it to say the use of unusual sets should be preceded by an understanding of their special operation. Read the directions for use; do not presume an adequacy of knowledge based on adaptation from other sets. They are not all alike.

Every set begins with a sturdy plastic piece having a sharp point called a spike (Figure 2.5). This spike is designed for insertion into the container closure. Sometimes the spike or the rubber stopper surface of the closure is lubricated to facilitate this insertion which, for the solid rubber stopper, may require considerable force. As mentioned earlier in the chapter, the spike may be fitted with an airway when no separate means of air ingress is provided in the bottle design. The configuration of the spike always should include a shield to prevent touch contamination as the set is being inserted in the bottle. Fingers should remain behind this shield at all times after the sterile protector is removed.

In sequence the next major structure usually is the drip chamber (Figure 2.5). It is an enlarged tube of plastic. The spike is fitted at its top and the set tubing exits from the bottom. Liquid flows from the spike into the chamber through the drip tube which is interposed between these

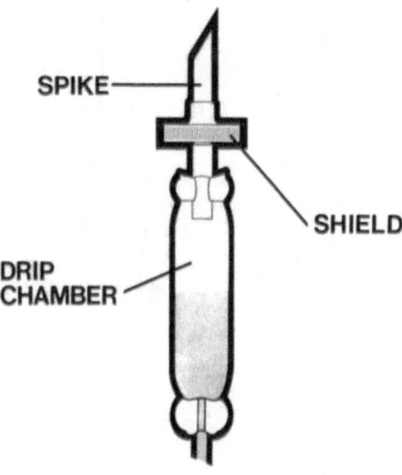

SPIKE

SHIELD

DRIP
CHAMBER

Figure 2.5

parts. Each manufacturer controls the diameter of the drip tube so the size of drops which form at its end can be converted by easy arithmetic into the volume of fluid being delivered (see Table 2.1). As an example, if the drip rate is 30 drops per minute in a set having a drip tube size which delivers 15 drops per milliliter, the infusion is flowing at 2 ml per minute or 120 ml per hour. Users should ascertain the standard for specific equipment upon first contact with it.

Table 2.1

	Drops/ml			
	Abbott	*Cutter*	*McGaw*	*Travenol*
Standard	15	20	15	10
Minidrip	60	50	60	60

When the set is primed, a fluid level is established in the lower part of the drip chamber. This level should be approximately midway between the end of the drip tube and the bottom of the drip chamber. If lower, the level will be insufficient to protect against entrainment of air in the fluid stream with the associated possibility of an air embolism. Levels at or near the drip tube will make it difficult to know fluid is moving in the set and at what rate it is moving. Priming usually is a very simple procedure because most drip chambers are flexible. With the downstream tubing occluded (by clamp or manually), the chamber is squeezed two or three times until a satisfactory level is established (Figure 2.6). Integral airway sets often will not require manipulation when a rigid fluid container is penetrated.

25

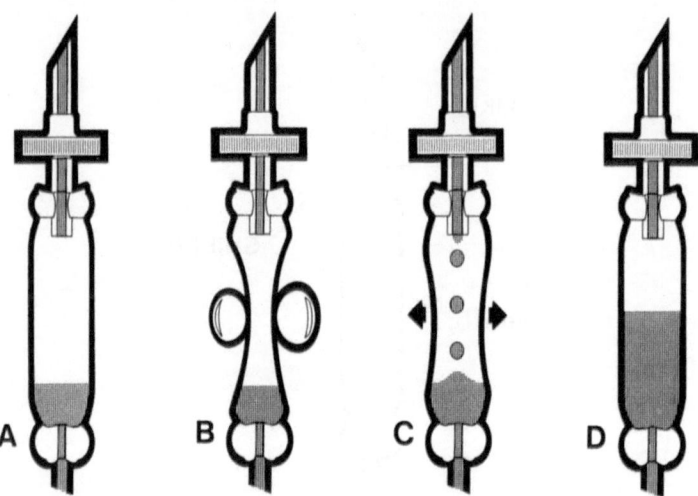

Figure 2.6 To prime a drip chamber, it is squeezed momentarily between the thumb and forefinger and then released. Prime level is approximately one half full

The fluid level will establish itself as the vacuum in the unit is relieved. If a mistake in use occurs and the drip chamber fluid becomes exhausted or the chamber flooded, some simple techniques can be employed to rectify the situation. Priming is complete when the fluid traverses the entire set, and no air is seen in the delivery tubing.

The simplest part of any administration set is the tubing, attached on one end to the drip chamber and on the other to a connector. Its length provides the patient some freedom of movement. The diameter of the tubing is relatively standard for each manufacturer. This size, whatever it is, has very little importance to the user. Because of its truly uncomplicated nature, tubing is rarely the source or site of any difficulties. In addition to serving as a conduit for fluid delivery, the administration set is intended to control the rate of infusion. Nearly every set has a rate controlling clamp which can be adjusted, so the infusion proceeds at different speeds in accordance with patient needs.

Two types of clamps are the most popular, the screw clamp and the roller clamp (Figure 2.7). Each has its devotees and supporters; the truth is they perform equally well. The screw clamp consists of plastic which encircles the delivery tube to occlude it gradually. The roller clamp has a wheel running along an inclined ramp. This wheel is fitted closer to the surface of the inclined plane at one end than the other, and the delivery tube passes through the space between the wheel and tube. As the wheel is turned, it imposes a tightening action against the tube and reduces flow. Many design variations have been claimed to be superior changes; none have yet proved to be so.

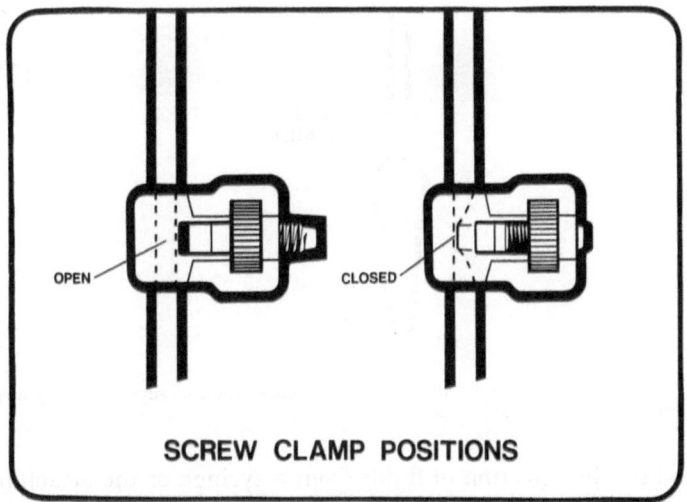

Figure 2.7a A screw clamp in both the open and closed position

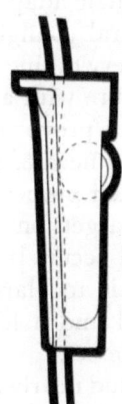

Figure 2.7b A roller clamp showing the tubing path under the roller

At the end of the set opposite from the drip chamber is the male (or occasionally female) Luer adapter. The Luer fitting has been adopted as the standard in many places in the world. Its dimensions are governed by agreement among engineers, making possible a satisfactory connection between parts from different manufacturing sources and the creation of a series of tubes and/or interlocked devices. These connections sometimes can be the source of leaks, as noted in a subsequent part of this chapter under the heading of Problems.

Additional features can be incorporated into a standard administration set to increase its flexibility. For instance, there are two devices which

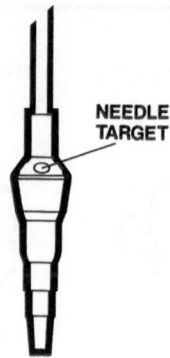

Figure 2.8 Flashball can be used as a site for administration of supplementary medication in some circumstances (see text)

accommodate the injection of fluids from a syringe or the attachment of an auxiliary set. These are the *Flashball* and the *Y* site.

The Flashball (Figure 2.8) nearly always is positioned between the end of the tubing and the Luer male adapter. It is formed of rubber and through the years has had several configurations. Basically, its lumen provides a conduit between delivery tubing and the Luer connector, while its rubber body is easy to puncture with a small needle (usually 22g or less). Originally it was used to 'prove' penetration of a vein. When squeezed after insertion of a steel needle, there is a 'flashback' of blood into the set if the needle is located properly. The most recent design of the Flashball has small circular targets on its surface intended to indicate where needle penetration should occur. If these reinforced locations are not used, or the needle gauge is too large, there is a possibility the Flashball rubber will not reseal and a leak will occur, particularly if unusual pressure develops in the set.

A *Y* site (Figure 2.9) can be found nearly anywhere in the set configuration.. There are a few custom design sets I have seen which include a *Y*

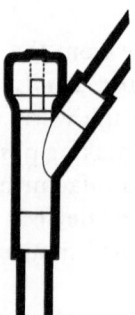

Figure 2.9 The Y site is a proper place for infusing medication in most instances

28

site immediately beneath the spike and upstream of the drip chamber. A common position is somewhere in the length of the set tubing. More than one Y site may be placed in a set. The device is made of a hard plastic body, formed as a Y, with one arm and the stem connected to the set tubing. The other arm is sealed by a resilient rubber diaphragm. Needles are passed through the diaphragm. Several design characteristics must be recognized in the use of the Y site and Flashball. Most important is that the rubber surfaces intended for needle penetration are not protected following sterilization (the spike and Luer connector ends are). Therefore, for each use the Y site must be carefully decontaminated to avoid carrying environmental organisms into the fluid path and directly into the patient. This statement does not mean a casual wipe of the part with a slightly damp alcohol sponge. A definitive decontamination routine should be followed, including the removal of foreign material and the application of an iodophor. Excess fluid should be removed with a sterile wipe. Then the part should be protected from touch or other contamination until the needly is inserted and removed. Since the surface is exposed to the environment constantly, the decontamination ritual should be practiced with each penetration of the rubber diaphragm.

There are a limited number of times the rubber body of the Flashball or the diaphragm of the Y site can be penetrated without impairing resealability. Therefore, this practice should be employed only occasionally. If additives are to be made regularly, other set configurations are more appropriate. An exception to this rule occurs when a Y site is punctured but the needle remains there for an extended period, as in the sequential flow set or special parenteral nutrition set (Figure 2.10).

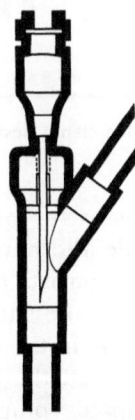

Figure 2.10 Needle penetrating Y site

29

Another option for the classic administration set is the micro-drip tube. Recall the drip tube is that part of the set structure which indicates flow by forming drops at its end. The size of the drops dictates a flow rate. In the micro-drip option the standard drip tube is replaced by one of much smaller diameter, usually a metal tube where the size can be controlled well. Small drops come from the end of such a tube. Therefore, control of fluid administration theoretically can be more accurate because quantities are subdivided into smaller parts. The advantage achieved by changing drip tube sizes is questionable, since control is mediated by the clamp; the drip tube is only a monitor. Micro-drip options are available in fully assembled sets or as an accessory which can be fitted into a standard set.

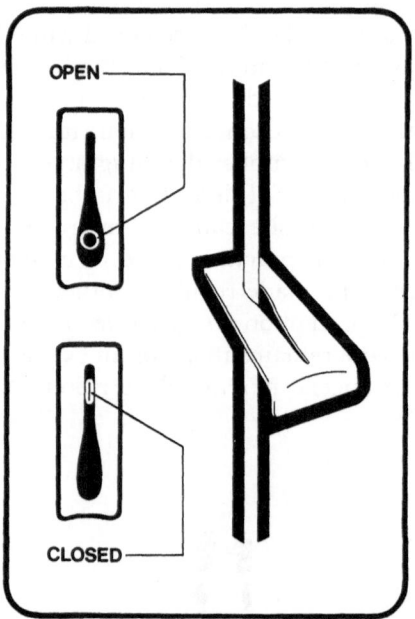

Figure 2.11 Slide clamp design and operation

Sometimes a second clamp is useful for the most efficient functioning of a special set design. A simple alternate to those described already is a slide clamp (Figure 2.11). It consists of a small rectangular piece of metal or plastic with a cutout in the shape of an elongated tear drop. Tubing is passed through the hole in the metal. As the slide is advanced to the narrow portion of the cutout, the lumen of the tube is gradually occluded until flow is interrupted completely. In actual practice the degree of flow control achieved by the slide clamp is less than in the roller or screw design. Therefore, the slide clamp is adapted best to on–off conditions rather than variations in partial flow.

There are a number of accessories which can be incorporated into the basic administration set. Some of these are shown in Figure 2.12.

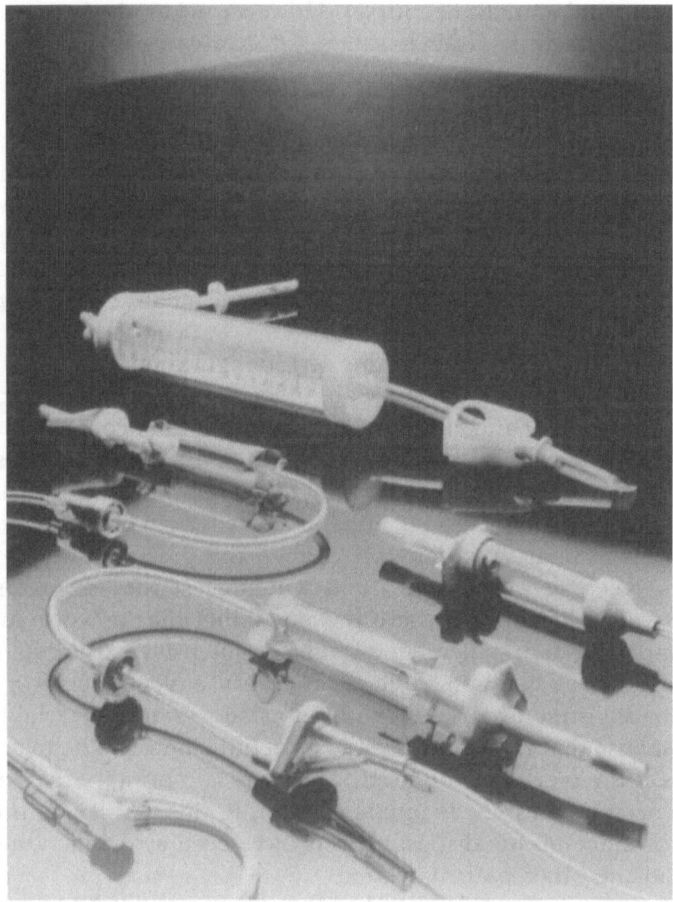

Figure 2.12 Several administration set accessories and alternate configurations for special purposes.

PROBLEMS

The administration set is a device of eminently simple design, but there are several interesting and sometimes troublesome problems which may develop during use. The most disconcerting is leakage. Since the set is designed to carry fluid from the container to the patient in a clean,

31

efficient manner, it is frustrating to find after assembly of the system that there is a leak. Even though the leak rate is only a few drops per several minutes, this quantity is enough for the patient to experience a feeling of water inundation when the bed and clothing become damp during the infusion. If the leak is at a connection in the system, the parts should be tightened, possibly precluding the need for further action (except changing the sheets and clothes, of course). However, when the leak is from a point which represents a defect in set manufacture, there is nothing which will remedy the situation short of changing the set. Tape, clamps, and other homemade potions are uniformly useless and dangerous.

The frequency of leaks which are the product of manufacturing faults is extremely low, except when a design or material defect is introduced inadvertently in otherwise successful mass production. It is a rare, forgiveable inconvenience (although it may not seem to be so at the time) when one considers the very low price paid (in terms of cents, not dollars – a real bargain in today's economy) for a sterile medical device that has so much utility.

When a Flashball is part of the set configuration and pressure is applied to the system to induce a rapid infusion, a separation may occur between the Flashball and either the tubing or the Luer connector. These parts are fitted together by 'friction', that is, their dimensions are designed in a way that makes the fit very tight between them. Most often no cement, glue or solvent is used to enhance the strength of the connection. A slight dimensional variation can change the pressure the joint will withstand. Keeping this fact in mind will suggest the use of a set *not* equipped with a Flashball if there is a possibility that pressure infusion will be employed as in emergency rooms or intensive care units.

Questions about function directed at nearly any physician or nurse having the slightest experience with infusion systems invariably will elicit a response that rate control is the most difficult attribute to achieve, regardless of the type of clamp used. There are two primary reasons why there has been no entirely adequate solution to this perplexing problem in the years since plastic disposable sets have been available. One is set related and the other patient related.

A characteristic of polyvinyl chloride tubing is the attribute of 'cold flow'. This term means the tube will tend to conform to a new shape at room temperature when certain forces are applied. Roller, screw and slide clamps impart such forces. Typically, there will be a diminution of flow over a period as short as 15–60 minutes for one setting of the clamp. A new setting intended to correct the problem will be followed by the same result. In frustration a final 'full open' setting may be adopted with the expectation it will be followed in due course by the diminishing flow seen before. No such luck! The infusion continues at the high rate (or even more) and the volume of liquid infused may be distressingly large. Many answers have been proposed, their validity usually documented by the inventor in an experiment which does not include the patient. No panacea for set clamps has been discovered or offered.

The second variable in flow rate control is the patient, notoriously more difficult to adjust and/or understand than any mechanical apparatus. The resistance to flow from a suspended fluid unit comes in part from patient venous pressure. As fluid from the container is infused, the liquid head pressure falls so the influence of venous pressure increases. When a

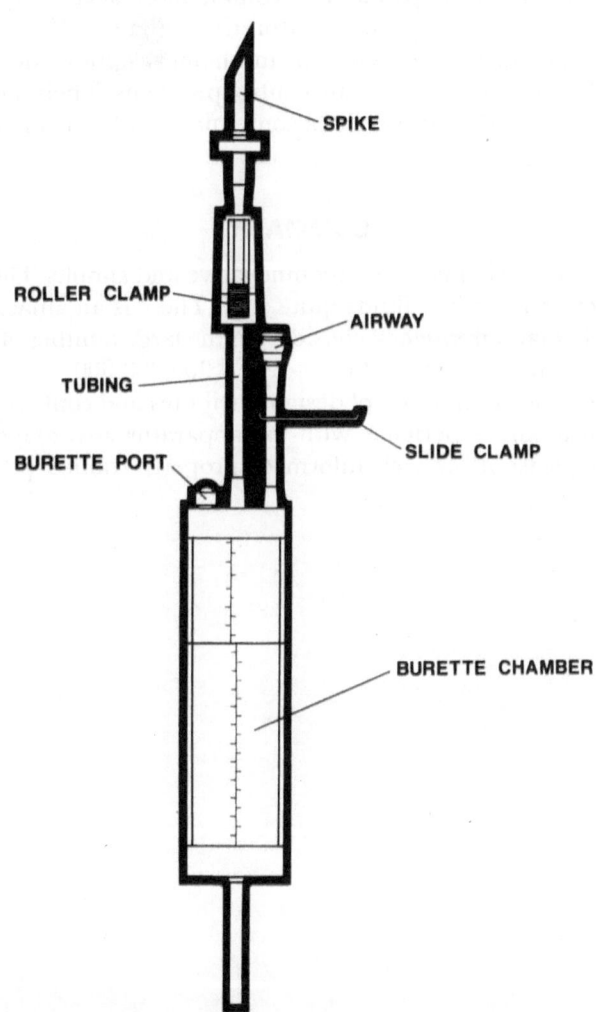

Figure 2.13 In line burette (see text Chapters 2 and 4)

patient changes position from that at which the infusion rate had been set, the venous pressure at the end of the set may change also. The initial position may be supine, followed by sitting and standing or walking. Little wonder it is that flow rate is so difficult to manage. For small children crying can raise the venous pressure to amazingly high limits and stop the infusion momentarily.

While there are other good reasons why flow rate control is difficult, these are the most important. If better control is mandatory for successful therapy, then users should select a pump or controller which meets the requirements of the intended application (see Chapter 8). To prevent excess infusion and perhaps monitor volume more accurately, a volume infusion chamber accessory (such as Buretrol – Figure 2.13) can be useful if a pump is not in the system. Non mechanical options do nothing to change the factors which cause rate control problems. Their only function is to prevent one of the most serious consequences of control failure, over infusion.

SUMMARY

Infusion system design is generally innovative and simple. The available products store and deliver fluids quite well. There is an amazingly small manufacturing fault frequency considering the large number of fluid units used in the United States alone – over 200,000,000 per year. User sensitivity for and recognition of design attributes and confounding problems can make any experience with the apparatus advantageous to the patient and pleasant for well informed, properly trained personnel.

3
Manufacturing

I do not anticipate any reader will indulge in the manufacture of large volume parenteral solutions based on the content of this chapter. (By definition, a large volume parenteral is more than 50 ml per unit. It is abbreviated LVP.) Rather I hope to demonstrate two important facts.

(1) There is sufficient complexity in the proper manufacture of these fluids to mandate that hospital pharmacies should not undertake the task.

(2) Parenteral solutions are no lesser drugs than most potent medicines. Manufacturers prepare them with great diligence and respect, and users should administer them with equal reverence and care. Compared to orally administered products where the gut forms a natural barrier, the intravascular route bypasses this protection completely and delivers drugs directly to the major transport system of the body without modification, detoxification or selection.

There are several general principles which define the procedures and environment for manufacture of large volume parenteral solutions. They are embodied in a regulation published by the United States Government called Good Manufacturing Practices, in statements by other governments, and in official compendia such as the *United States Pharmacopeia*, the *British Pharmacopoeia*, and the *European Pharmacopeia*.

The basic guidance provided by these several sources can be summarized as follows:

(1) The manufacturing environment is clean and well maintained.

(2) During solution preparation several appropriate tests are performed to monitor the process. Each batch must pass these tests.

(3) Records for the batch are developed and analyzed to show adequate procedures were followed and the resulting solution is within narrow ranges of permissible variation.

35

The ultimate solution product must meet rigid criteria for patient use. Generally stated, these characteristics are:

(1) Sterile,
(2) non-pyrogenic,
(3) nearly particle free,
(4) chemically correct, and
(5) properly labeled

At the very minimum, testing for these attributes must be done when *each* batch or lot of solution is completed. The results must be evaluated and recorded before release of the solution for patient use.

To adhere to the requirements noted above and still make available an inexpensive product in exceedingly large quantities (the total use of large volume parenteral solutions in the United States in 1982 was over 200,000,000 units), commercial manufacturers have developed efficient procedures that result in reliable product output on a regular basis. The important aspects of their technology are described in the following paragraphs.

RAW MATERIALS

There are two basic components in every large volume parenteral solution, the solutes and the solvent. Almost without exception the solvent is water; it makes up more than 98% of the solution and will be discussed later in the chapter. The solutes are chemicals of various types ranging from simple materials such as salt (sodium chloride) and sugar (dextrose) to more complex substances such as alcohol, amino-acetic acid (glycine), and mixtures of amino acids. Each of these is purchased with a demand to the seller that special criteria for chemical purity be met so as to make the substances medically suitable. Sources of raw materials are not checked simply by testing incoming shipments. Their sites and procedures of manufacture are evaluated routinely by personal visit from the LVP solution vendor and in several other ways. Failure to meet rigid standards often means temporary or permanent loss of the opportunity to sell to large volume parenteral solution producers.

Transportation of the raw materials to the manufacturer is an important point. It is unsuitable to use a tank car or a reusable drum which may have carried toxic substances in a previous shipment because these bulk containers cannot be cleansed adequately. Special arrangements are made by manufacturers to guarantee the proper selection of conveyance apparatus.

Upon arrival at the solution manufacturing site a battery of tests are applied to the raw materials which is intended to demonstrate the product is within specification and does not contain undesirable extra substances.

Only after meeting these testing specifications successfully does the raw material become available for use in solution preparation. Then the raw material is labeled and stored in a location known to be suitable to its chemistry until it is used.

EQUIPMENT

Apparatus must be very large to manufacture solutions in batch sizes of 10,000 to 25,000 liters (2650–6600 US gallons). In addition it must be adaptable to several different temperatures, easily cleaned, absolutely corrosion resistant and nearly completely dismountable for inspection purposes. It must benefit from expert maintenance at all times; even the smallest malfunction is intolerable. A final requirement is that it be suitable for the prescribed manufacturing tasks to which it will be applied. *Ad hoc* adaptation and innovation are not laudable performance criteria in this aspect of the solution manufacturing business, as they can lead to unanticipated difficulties for which testing barriers are not included in the normal safeguard mechanism.

PERSONNEL

People are the most important component of the manufacturing environment. They must be well trained; each individual must feel a responsibility for insuring the health of his/her fellow man. Workers at all levels should be sensitive to the possibility of equipment malfunction or other unexpected events which may have even the slightest possibility of leading to an aberration in product integrity.

In order to perform well each person must know his/her duties. The work to be done must be documented in specifications and training manuals so that it can be understood by new people.

Constant attention to immaculate personal hygiene is critical. It is not enough that all workers in the proximity of solution manufacture be dressed in clothing designed to protect the product from the worker (not *vice versa*). Nearly any clothing barrier can be thwarted by carelessness and lack of cleanliness. Manufacturers spend many thousands of dollars in teaching proper techniques for simple tasks like hand washing, even though the washed hands moments later will be covered by powder free gloves.

All of these precautions and preparations should lead to workers who have pride in the product they make. Every person involved in solutions manufacture must sense they have an important role.

SOLUTION PREPARATION

The first step in the development of a solution batch is mixing all the solutes into the solvent liquid. Most often the water (the solvent) is pumped from special wells drilled to 1000 feet or more; occasionally potable water from a city system is used. Whatever the source, water is tested daily. If it fails to meet rigid standards, it cannot be used for solution. Correction of the deficiency must be made before it can become a raw material.

Two elements for which daily tests are crucial are micro-organism population and pyrogenicity. These factors can alter the quality of the final product significantly; faults may go undiscovered if measurements are not made early in the manufacturing sequence.

The quality and transport of solutes, various chemicals which when mixed with the water convert it to formulations typically prescribed by physicians, have been discussed in the preceding paragraphs on raw materials. At the time of solution preparation they are weighed or measured in some other acceptable way and placed in the water. The weighing/measuring is usually done by one person, verified by another, and confirmed by a printed report from whatever device is used. Before the solution mixture is released to the next part of the process, some chemical tests are performed to verify the accuracy of the mixing procedure. This step is the first of many similar to it which continually reconfirm the content of the formulation.

After all of the testing results are received, a senior official of the plant authorizes release of the batch to the filling sequence. Filling is the process in which the bulk solution is subdivided into individual units and placed in containers suitable for use in patient care. Techniques are adapted to some extent from the food and drink industry but have been polished considerably to reduce contamination and sustain the quality of the carefully prepared bulk.

The primary apparatus is the filling machine, an automated mechanism which measures precisely the stipulated quantity of liquid and places it in a container. In its useful life the machine must perform this task reliably millions of times. For instance, it would be unforgivable if different solution units had a highly variably volume. The user would find such unpredictability intolerable in rendering proper patient care.

Glass containers, before they pass through the filling machine, are inspected for integrity and basic cleanliness. A suitable sample of every shipment is checked for proper dimensions. After receipt from the manufacturer the glass is washed and rinsed thoroughly. Above all it is handled gently to avoid chips and cracks which would enhance the risk of subsequent fluid contamination by unintentional ingress of microorganisms.

Plastic containers are usually made by the solution manufacturer, as compared to glass containers which almost always come from a geographically distant glass plant. The plastic either is extruded and sealed or molded carefully and then stored in a protected environment. A rinsing procedure may be necessary before use.

A closure apparatus for glass or plastic must be assembled separately from the main container body. Various raw materials making up the closure are checked for dimensional accuracy, subjected to cleaning just before use, and protected while awaiting final fitting into the container. The glass container closure is much more complex than for most plastic units. The amount of handling necessary for plastic units is considerably less, another of the many desirable features of plastic.

The glass container closure is fixed in position after a vacuum has been drawn on the unit by a capping machine. The presence of this vacuum at the time of use is judged by many to be an indication of likely sterility. It is uncertain after these many years exactly how reliable this indicator is. Several units have been found in which a vacuum was present but a leak followed by contamination had occurred nevertheless.

Sterilization of essentially all large volume parenteral solutions having a water solvent is by terminal heat. (There are a few exceptions which are not worthy of note and embody an undesirable risk of non-sterility in my opinion.) The heat is supplied as steam which is one of the most efficient heat transfer mechanisms available. To determine that a reliable sterilization sequence has occurred, the generally accepted standard is a combined measure of time and temperature, called an integrated heat history. It is nothing more than a mathematical transformation of time and temperature into a factor which can be related to the probability of sterility. In the most up to date nomenclature, the measure of proper sterilization is in the form of the likelihood of non-sterility (or risk of a unit not being sterile). It is common practice to use a heating process which will produce a risk of non-sterility not greater than 1 unit per 1,000,000 produced. Actually, all manufacturers seem to be better than this level of performance with a considerable margin of safety.

A few solutions are known to be heat sensitive. These receive a smaller integrated heat history justified by risk–benefit judgments for the patient use of the formulation.

It is no longer satisfactory to heat every type of solution in a sterilizer set to deliver the same amount of steam for the same time, regardless of solution formulation, unit size, quantity being sterilized and many other factors. A complete understanding of the sterilization process must be attained before proper sterility goals can be described and achieved. Likewise, the mechanical performance of the sterilizer vessel and its controls and the quality of the steam produced must be included in any comprehensive estimate of solution quality. In recent years there have been examples in both the United States and the United Kingdom of faults in the sterilization process which have ended in patient deaths. In these instances a better understanding of the sterilization process would have avoided a serious clinical problem.

The last manufacturing steps in the solution preparation sequence are packaging, storage and shipping. Individual units are placed in protective cartons so they can be stored and shipped without damage. Storage should be in conditions which will not impair product quality. Temperature is confined to reasonable ranges. Cleanliness of the warehouse is important. Clear labelling of the cartons is necessary. Here also the lighter weight, much less fragile plastic container has a superiority over glass. These aspects of the glass/plastic comparison cannot be ignored.

The final step in the process is testing. Many people believe it is this part of solution preparation which guarantees that no harm will come to the patient. Nothing could be farther from the truth. In actual fact the number of samples selected at the end of manufacture to evaluate sterility and non-pyrogenicity is too small to detect any low level contaminant. Only the gross type of sterility fault can be found with the standard United States Pharmacopeia (USP) test. Tests for chemistry tend to be more helpful in discovering errors because the causes of such difficulty rarely select out a small number of units. The real assurance of quality is not testing but a full understanding and absolute control of the manufacturing process. A quotation often repeated by knowledgeable people is 'Product quality is inherent in the process, not the test'. Liberally translated – 'you can't test product quality in'.

SUMMARY

Large volume parenteral solution manufacturers prepare products by reliable, well engineered mass production methods. The solutions have a high quality and long stability. They are eminently reliable pharmaceutical products, even considering extremely rare lapses in quality which have been demonstrated in the last decade. These products should not be made locally (in hospital).

Parenteral solutions are a bargain. They are made rigorously, essentially guaranteed by the manufacturer until use, shipped throughout the world, and (in the United States at least), all for usually less than one dollar for one liter.

4

Proper Use of
Infusion Systems

The purpose of this chapter is to describe the assembly of equipment for an intravenous infusion, initiation of the infusion procedure and its termination, and some variables which result from inserting optional devices in the system.

Here is a convenient way to remember the fundamental elements of a successful infusion. The Three C's – **contamination, compatibility** and **complexity**. Having a constant sensitivity for each of these factors will result in good infusion practices. The first C – contamination – refers to anything (everything) leading to the ingress of environmental micro-organisms which can be infused subsequently into the patient or multiply in the system and then enter the bloodstream. The second – compatibility – concerns inappropriate mixing of incompatible ingredients or components in an infusion system. Complexity – the third C – is a reminder that complicated systems may produce unexpected consequences.

From these words come a sign which should be posted in every patient care area:

COMMANDMENTS OF GOOD INFUSION PRACTICE

AVOID CONTAMINATION
BE CERTAIN OF COMPATIBILITIES
DIMINISH COMPLEXITY

The simplest of intravenous infusions involves the administration of fluid and/or electrolyte replacement solution into a vein using the force of gravity as the propelling energy, controlling the rate with an inexpensive plastic clamp, and gaining vascular access by means of inserting a steel needle into a peripheral vein. Equipment and supplies necessary to accomplish this therapy are

(1) A fluid filled reservoir which can preserve sterility and non-pyrogenicity during storage following manufacture,

(2) An administration set with a standard drip chamber and at least 60″ ($\simeq 1.5$ m) of tubing which terminates in a needle adapter,

(3) A steel needle, 1–1½″ (2.5–4 cm) long and 20 gauge internal diameter,

(4) A tourniquet,

(5) Antiseptic solution impregnated in an applicator, and

(6) Tape.

The first action is to identify the patient to whom the fluid is to be given, and verify the label on the container has the same name and hospital number as the patient. The next step is to compare the stated content of the container with the physician's order being executed. These activities are important because they insure the right patient is getting the correct solution. No container should be in an active infusion system unless it is labeled with a patient name and number. Even if no admixtures have been made and the solution has been taken directly from floor stock, the recipient name and hospital number must be shown on the label. Only in this way can persons other than the individual who initiates the infusion be certain at a later time the correct fluid is being administered.

Before 'spiking' a flexible plastic fluid container, squeeze it two or three times, moving your hands after each maneuver. Look for leaks particularly at the heat sealed seams or near the ports. If a glass container is being used, check its content for clarity and apparent purity. You should see nothing but crystal clear, sparkling water. Look carefully for cracks in the glass, usually at the base or neck of the bottle. If a defect is detected, discard the container and select another which meets your criteria for adequate quality.

The following steps are appropriate to mount the administration set in a flexible plastic container.

(1) Place the container on a clean uncluttered surface.

(2) Open the wrapping for the administration set, unwind the tubing, and move the clamp to a closed position.

(3) Remove the protector from the spike on the end of the drip chamber and afterward treat the exposed surface as sterile. Do not use an antiseptic solution.

(4) Remove the protector from the administration port of the flexible container. No antiseptic solution should be applied.

(5) With a slight twisting motion insert the spike into the port until a bevel on the spike prevents further penetration. The spike must be the full distance into the port in order to have traversed the membrane which is integral in the port assembly.

(6) Hang the container on a stand so there is at least 36 inches (one meter) of distance between the bottom of the drip chamber and the apparent heart level of the patient (*see* later discussion).

Prime the drip chamber by squeezing it once or twice so approximately one half of the total chamber volume is occupied by fluid. Always leave 1–1½ inches (2.5–4.0 centimeters) between the end of the drip tube and the fluid level to visualize the rate of flow easily. Open the clamp slowly and observe fluid run into the tubing until it reaches the needle adapter; then close the clamp. Do not remove the protector. Place the filled tubing in a location where it will be easily accessible when the venipuncture is completed.

If a rigid, air-dependent container is being used, only step (5) above changes significantly as follows:

(5) With a slight twisting motion, insert the spike into the proper location on the rubber stopper. If the bottle has a separate airway, squeeze the drip chamber of the administration set and release as the container is being inverted. When an integral airway set is being used, invert the bottle without manipulating the drip chamber.

The next step involves preparing the patient, mentally and physically, for the venipuncture. When this venipuncture is the first to be experienced by the patient, a few moments of explanation will go a long way to relieve anxiety. If it is one in a long series, the patient probably knows more then you do. Whatever the situation, the dominant theme is empathy. Put your self in the position of the patient. Would you enjoy seeing a venipuncturist shaking like a leaf and lacking any sense of confidence? Would you accept an individual with unclean hands? Would you submit to multiple penetrations of the needle done carelessly or to a single entry through the skin followed by prolonged searching for the vein with the needle? Would you allow a person with a dirty uniform or scraggly hair hanging in their face (like a sheepdog?) to perform a venipuncture? I would not! Avoid these and other obvious 'turnoffs'. The most painful part of a patient's hospital stay can be intravenous infusion and blood sampling experiences. Do your best to make them less than memorable.

Select a site for the venipuncture. Some 'experts' advise the use of the most distal peripheral vein possible, anticipating there will be many more episodes and planning to move proximally for successive needle insertions. Often this dictum is translated to an attempt to cannulate a barely visible distal phalangeal vein. If successfully penetrated, the likelihood is small of it remaining viable without infiltration throughout the infusion. The proper procedure is as follows:

Select a venipuncture site

(1) Which can be decontaminated properly and effectively,

(2) Where there is a reasonable chance of a successful puncture at the first attempt,

(3) In a location that can accommodate anchoring of the needle, and

(4) So the patient will be comfortable throughout the infusion.

If a finger or hand vein meets these criteria in your opinion, proceed. If not, make a more reasonable choice.

You may wish to raise a vein temporarily, making it more visible by distending it with blood, to assess the wisdom of your judgement. This step is performed by applying a tourniquet above the chosen location and waiting for the vein to fill. Sometimes placing the arm in a more dependent posture relative to the heart will hasten the process. When you are satisfied, remove the tourniquet.

If you believe there is too much hair at and surrounding the place you intend to penetrate the skin, clip it with a scissors. Shaving abrades the surface and leaves nicks and gashes which are potential portals for infection. Apply an antiseptic solution, and let it dry for the prescribed time. Thereafter, do not touch the area with unsterile utensils or your fingers. Tighten the tourniquet again, remembering you are seeking only to occlude superficial venous return, not all of the arterial and venous structures of the arm. Be gentle. Move rapidly after taking this step so the patient does not experience undue and prolonged discomfort from venous engorgement of the arm.

Open the needle package and expose the hub. Then remove the protector from the administration set needle adapter and marry the two firmly. Extract the needle from its container. (Some people wear sterile gloves after this point but I think these accoutrements are more 'show' than useful.) After placing a light counter pressure on the skin surface along the axis of the vein, insert the needle through the skin with the bevel up.

There are several acceptable techniques for what follows. You will see them demonstrated successfully from time to time. One method that is used frequently is to proceed directly toward the vein. When it is entered, there will be a 'flash' of blood in the administration set tubing. Then, thread the needle into the vein a short distance. Remove the tourniquet. Open the clamp slowly and observe the onset of flow into the vein with a sense of triumph and accomplishment. Another approach is to penetrate the skin, aiming at a site adjacent to the vein. Tilt the needle slightly, capture the vein wall and advance the needle into the vein lumen. Those who prefer this method believe the two step approach results in more successes because the venipuncturist can concentrate on vein penetration without concern at the same moment for entering the skin.

When an over the needle catheter is being inserted, the technique is approximately the same as for a steel needle except that another maneuver is needed in which the needle is withdrawn while the plastic cannula remains. Anchoring the needle or catheter with tape should be done after fluid is running well (*see* below). More tape does not translate to a more secure arrangement. One piece across the hub usually is sufficient for a needle. It should be wide to have enough adhesive surface to be useful. It should not cover the point of skin penetration. Another length of tape should be applied to anchor the administration set to the skin, leaving the distance between the needle hub and the tape quite loose. This section of the set is a strain relief. It will protect (to some extent) against disruption of the venipuncture if some unexpected pull of the tubing occurs. Tape never should encircle the arm completely.

The venipuncture normally needs no dressing or other protection. If it is covered, some adverse local development may be overlooked because it is not immediately apparent. Very recently transparent dressings have become popular and some hospitals have instituted a routine practice of covering the venipuncture with a 2"–3" square of this material. This procedure is expensive and adds nothing, in my opinion, to the safety of an infusion. There are no convincing facts to support this approach to infusion technology. When the venipuncture is complete, the date, time, and size of needle should be written on the tape.

When the needle or catheter is in the vein securely, flow rate can be established by manipulating the set clamp to occlude the tubing lumen partially. The initial setting will require adjustment, more often in the early phases of the infusion. Visit the patient's bedside frequently and adjust the clamp according to your observations. If the patient moves to a chair, it will be necessary to change the clamp adjustment because the venous pressure at the end of the needle will have changed. Similarly, following ambulation the flow rate will need modulation.

The most dangerous malfunction of a gravity infusion system is a 'runaway' which occurs when a substantial amount of fluid unintentionally enters the patient in a short time. This event ushers in the possibility of overwhelming the cardiovascular system and causing acute failure. The disaster can be avoided by checking the infusion frequently in order to catch a 'runaway' in its incipient phase.

When assuming responsibility for an infusion in progress, for instance at change of shifts or transfer of a patient, you should check its status completely including verification of the patient identity with the container label, container content with the physician order, flow rate concordance with label statement and condition of the venipuncture site. This complete survey will establish a mental picture for you of the therapy being administered.

Almost every infusion consists of more than one container of solution. Therefore, there will be a need to change containers, perhaps more than once. The process is simple. When the administration set spike is extracted from the nearly empty container, care must be exercised to avoid touch contaminating the spike before it is seated in the next container. Even though the new container is at the bedside, the full ritual of identification should be followed. No assumption should be made for correctness of a colleague's work or work ready product.

Several parenteral drugs are given intermittently. These include antibiotics, some antitumor agents, and miscellaneous medication. To facilitate the orderly administration of these drug containing parenteral fluids, several products of the same general type have been developed.

The typical apparatus which is used now to administer one dose of intermittent parenteral medication, other than a short (bolus) dose, relies upon differential pressures created between two containers raised to different heights above the patient. The drug container is called the primary (my nomenclature) and it is the higher of the two units (remember the nomenclature by thinking of highest, first, primary). (*see* Figure 4.1). The secondary unit contains a common parenteral solution such as 5% dextrose or saline. In selecting the secondary solution, avoid a formula which will result in an interaction with the drug. To create the pressure differential, the secondary unit is positioned below the primary using a hanger of adequate length which is supplied with the administration set. To assure complete emptying of the primary container before the secondary automatically begins supplying fluid for infusion, the lowest part of the primary unit must be above the highest point of the secondary.

The principle on which these two container, intermittent 'single shot'

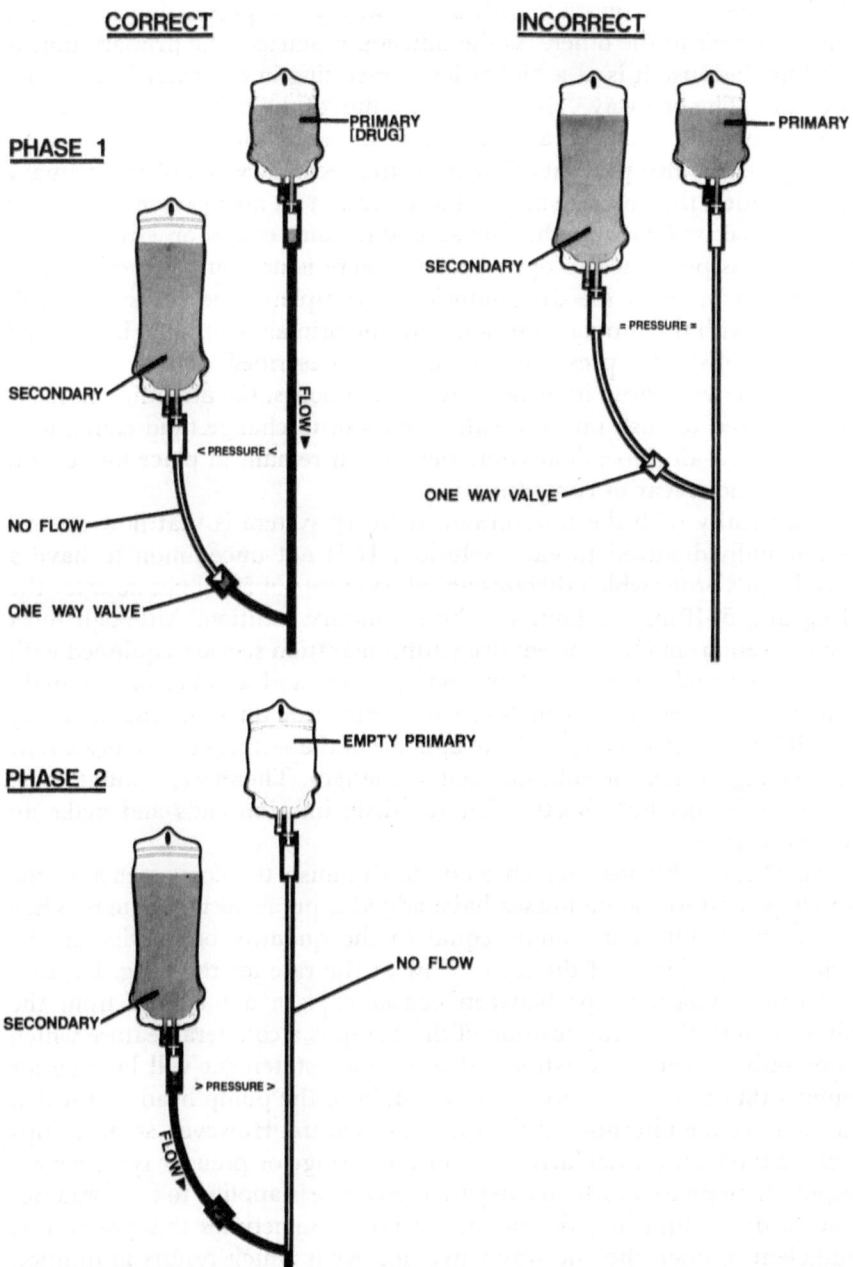

Figure 4.1 Left side of the drawing depicts the two phases of fluid administration from an intermittent drug administration system. The right side (which is an incorrect configuration) shows the primary and secondary containers hung at the same level, a circumstance which will prevent sequential flow

47

devices operates is gravity with a one way valve preventing flow from one container to the other. As the infusion is started, the primary unit is 'on line' because it is at a higher level, resulting in a greater hydrostatic pressure. The one way valve prevents reflux of the primary solution into the secondary container, and the same pressure which closes the valve to stop reflux also prevents flow from the secondary. Until the primary unit empties, the pressure in its administration set always remains higher than the secondary branch. The secondary unit comes on stream when the valve is permitted to open because there is no counterforce to close it. At that moment the drug infusion is complete, and the system will continue with the support solution until the primary container is replaced to re-establish the pressure relationships described above. Since the interval between drug infusions often is 3–8 hours, the attending nurse is not required to rush into the patient's room to change fluid containers. Being a non-air dependent container, it can remain in place for several hours without fear of contamination.

A difficulty with the intermittent delivery system is that flow control is not individualized to each solution. It is not uncommon to have a physician's order which dictates an infusion rate of 50 ml per hour for the drug and 5–10 ml per hour for the secondary solution. Although most configurations of intermittent drug administration sets are equipped with clamps for each arm or a clamp on one arm and another on the main line, the various factors which influence flow rate often interact in a way to mitigate the necessary delicate balance of the settings to achieve a flow rate change when the solution source changes. Therefore, a nurse must come to the bedside shortly after the drug infusion ends and make an adjustment.

To obviate this visit which tends to diminish the convenience of the entire procedure, some nurses have added a pump to the system. They set the total infusion volume equal to the quantity of solution in the primary container and the initial flow at the rate for the drug. Because the height relationships between containers are not altered from the above description, interposition of the pump is a collateral feature which adds only a fancy downstream clamp. This statement will be true for pumps that rely on gravity to deliver fluid to the pump head and which do *not* have the intermittent fill and draw feature. However, some pumps (*see* Chapter 8), particularly those of the syringe or plunger type, have a rapid filling phase in which a negative pressure is applied to the container line to draw fluid into the pump reservoir. Sometimes this pressure is sufficient to open the one way valve, an event which results in dilution of the drug solution with fluid from the secondary container. If this unanticipated action occurs on every stroke, there will be drug remaining in the primary container when the fluid volume counter on the pump is satisfied. The rate will change, but all the drug will not have been infused. It will continue, now at a slower pace, and the intention of intermittent delivery may be thwarted.

This instance is one of many which can occur when substantially different parts of infusion apparatus normally not intended for each other, are connected together. The universal compatibility of Luer connectors and other fittings provides a temptation to assemble disposable equipment and hardware which may not function together properly. Merely because tubes can be married without a leak does not mean they should be connected. Always analyze the likely result of your 'invention' if you are straying from the proven path. Demonstrate to yourself and others the safety, reliability, and effectiveness of the system before applying it in patient care.

A second common variation of the most simple infusion system configuration is the inclusion of one or more 'Y' sites in the administration set tubing. These are plastic pieces which have one limb of the 'Y' connected to the tubing and the other covered by a latex rubber diaphragm (see Chapter 2). The main stem of the 'Y' is connected to tubing which ends in the needle adapter or Luer fitting. The purpose of this piece is to facilitate injections of additional substances by providing a resealable surface (the latex rubber) which can be decontaminated properly before each use. Some sets, often favored by anesthesiologists, have multiple 'Y' sites distributed at various locations throughout the length of the set tubing. Rarely is this arrangement needed during general floor care of the patient. Not only is this configuration confusing but also it encourages the administration of different substances simultaneously or sequentially which may not be chemically compatible. The multiple 'Y' site set is more dangerous than useful except in very unique circumstances, as it encourages infusion equipment configurations which can induce human error.

The correct use of a 'Y' site is a simple procedure involving primarily proper decontamination of the latex surface. Application of an iodophor followed by the prescribed brief drying period is the approved method. Some people use an alcohol swab which is time honored but less effective. It is often more ritual than real. There is merit in exercising some vigor in the decontamination effort, since between uses the 'Y' site surface is exposed to unknown insults and perils of the environment which must be cleaned completely before the 'Y' site is safe again for penetration.

The needle which penetrates the latex diaphragm preferably should be 22 gauge or smaller and never larger than a 20 gauge. If this admonition is ignored, there is a chance of 'coring' the rubber or making a hole which will not reseal when the needle is withdrawn.

The final step before making an injection through a 'Y' site is to occlude the tubing 'upstream', the portion connected to the other limb of the 'Y'. Failure to do so will allow whatever is being injected to flow in both directions, into the patient and into the fluid container which results in improper drug delivery. If drug and fluid are to be given simultaneously, the 'Y' site method is not suitable. The needle is never allowed to remain in the 'Y' site in anticipation of another use. When the infusion is done, it is removed. For long term continuous administration of supplementary medication or fluids, a 'Y' site port is not proper or safe since it can be the source of direct contamination of the administration set and fluid passing through it.

An accessory which has become very popular because it fits well into central admixture programs is the 'minibag', a fluid container holding 50–100ml. Small glass bottles are also available for the same purpose but are used rarely. The minibag is a miniature large volume parenteral fluid container with an administration set port and additive port of conventional size and configuration. Usually it is prepared in the pharmacy by injecting a drug through the admixture port. Often diluting fluid is already present. The system remains sealed to the intrusion of outside elements because it is non-air dependent, the admixture port reseals, and the administration set port has not been transgressed. A proper label is affixed in the pharmacy.

Upon arrival in the patient care area the minibag should be placed in the drug repository in a refrigerator, unless cooling is prohibited specifically by a statement on the label. When the time comes for administration, the bag is processed in the usual manner by taking it to the patient's bedside, verifying the potential recipient's identity and compliance with the physician's order, and placing it in the infusion system. A minibag is frequently the drug container mounted in an intermittent delivery system described above.

A volume control fluid reservoir, often called a 'buretrol' because it has similarities to a burette found in a chemistry laboratory, is used commonly in infusion systems but seems to be losing popularity. It is a dangerous device, in my opinion, because it encourages practices which transgress good techniques emphasized throughout this book. The buretrol (see Figure 2.13) is a cylinder of about 6 inches (15 centimeters) in length and 1 inch (2·5 centimeters) in diameter, with volume markings on the side. There are many variations provided by several different manufacturers. The most simple has a short 'pigtail' tubing with a clamp at the top which ends in an administration set spike that can be inserted in a fluid reservoir. There is a latex covered port on the top cover also which will admit a needle. At the bottom is a float valve which remains open until fluid no longer is present in the cylinder. There is a suitable length of tubing leading away from the buretrol which forms an administration set, or the buretrol can be connected into a set.

To use the buretrol after it is connected to a fluid container, the clamp is opened after the downstream clamp is closed. Filling occurs to the desired level, and the fluid supply then is shut off. The downstream clamp is opened to deliver the desired flow rate which is followed and controlled more readily than when administration is directly from a minibag or large volume parenteral fluid container because the volume markings on the side of the container provide an accurate frame of reference.

When a buretrol is used to administer a drug, the concentrated agent is placed in the cylinder through the latex port with a needle and syringe. Then the total volume of fluid is raised to the prescribed level, and the infusion is initiated. When the buretrol is empty, the drug has been given.

Problems associated with burette type devices are the Three C's once again.

The potential for initial contamination derives from difficulty in decontaminating the latex diaphragm and its frequent re-use for multiple additives. Once inside, organisms can proliferate in many places, sliding into the solution as they do so. Careless management of buretrols results in leaving them in infusion arrangements for long periods of time. Because of the greater inherent danger of contamination, they and the entire system should be changed every 24 hours.

If there are physician's orders for several different drugs (perhaps two antibiotics and a cardiac medication) the temptation to place them in the buretrol in sequence is strong. This action may be taken by unsuspecting people without regard to the potential for incompatibilities between the agents. Because there are residuals of previously completed infusions in the cylinder when the new drug is inserted, an incompatibility may occur covertly or overtly. This reaction can create undesirable particulates or even worse, diminish or eradicate the potency of a drug. When the anticipated clinical action does not materialize, the physician may conclude the drug is ineffective and make an inappropriate change in therapy. If a burette device is used to administer drugs, only one agent should be placed in the cylinder. When more than one drug is to be administered, other arrangements should be made.

I have described only the simplest of buretrols. Many different designs are available. For instance, there is one with a filter at the bottom rather than a valve. Sometimes the filter becomes clogged partially ('loaded' – see Chapter 7) and subsequently flow rate is difficult to control. Another type can be fixed for a straight infusion where the buretrol acts as a drip chamber. To function in this manner various clamps and tubes must be set properly. These complexities can and occasionally will lead to malfunction of the infusion system, and the consequence of malfunction is patient risk and diminished patient care quality.

I see little value in the use of burette type devices. Every reasonable activity which can be performed with them can be accomplished safely and easily by another, better product which in most instances is less expensive than a burette.

SUMMARY

Infusion systems can be set up and operated with ease and safety. If the equipment selected is simple, the task will not be onerous. If the amount of attention given to the infusion by the responsible individual is adequate, the procedure will be safe for the patient. If common rules are observed, the result will be efficacious as intended by the physician.

5

Organization of an I.V. Service

In this chapter I will describe an operation orientated organization within the hospital to obtain, store, dispense properly, label, deliver and administer large volume (and some small volume) parenteral solutions and associated drugs to patients. This organization, which I consider optimal, does not exist anywhere to my knowledge. It includes certain technologies which are emerging now from research and development. Therefore, the contents of the chapter may be termed a 'vision of the future'. I believe this future is not far off. Pharmacists who cannot envisage adoption of all elements of this program should seek to accommodate those which seem most appropriate immediately and prepare for other components somewhat later.

The organization recognizes the mandated responsibility of many interacting groups in hospitals. Duties are assigned with a view to obtaining the highest level of expertise for the management of a critical function. Involvement of medical staff committees, nursing staff leaders and administration personnel is the key to the ultimate success of this program. Table 5.1 delineates the major actions which are attendant upon the successful use of parenteral solutions and related disposables in any hospital. The group judged to be most responsible for routine and regular implementation of these actions is also shown.

A slightly different schema would pertain for handling the hardware which is making increasing inroads into the administration of intravenous solutions. These products would include pumps, controllers, mechanical clamps and monitoring devices.

53

Table 5.1 Management of drugs and disposables

Action	Responsibility
Specifications of product content and performance	P&T committee – Medical staff Chief pharmacist*
Purchase	Purchasing – Administration
Receipt of product	Pharmacy
Storage of product	Pharmacy
Initiation of order for dispensing	Attending physician
Dispensing and labelling	Pharmacy
Delivery	(1) Pharmacy controlled service (2) Automated systems
Administration to patient (initial)	Clinical pharmacist i.v. Administration team
Administration (monitoring)	Clinical pharmacist Staff nurse
Adverse effect detection	All personnel
Adverse effect analysis	Attending physician P&T committee Clinical pharmacist

* May be delegated to an assistant
P&T refers to the Pharmacy and Therapeutics committee

Table 5.2 Management of hardware

Action	Responsibility
Specifications and Performance needs	P&T committee – Medical staff Critical care physician
Durability	Bioengineer
Disposable parts	Clinical pharmacist Nurse*
Purchase	Purchasing – Administration
Receipt	Asset clerk
Use	Clinical pharmacist i.v. Administration team Staff nurse
Maintenance	Bioengineer

* Often a nurse capable in this discipline is not available or apparent. No person should be appointed 'just to have a nurse'.

Reporting relationships for administrative purposes are important to the functional success of this system. The following diagram delineates

54

the lines of command that will implement the proposed system best in my opinion:

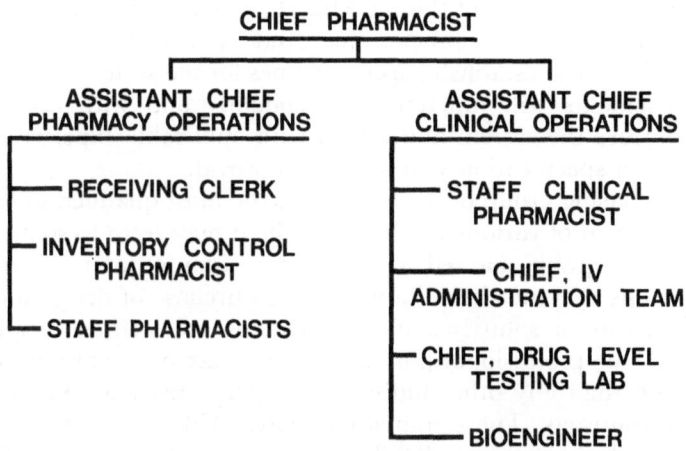

Obviously, the proposed system is a radical departure from what is now commonplace. It might be argued that less changes from current tradition will make adaptation easier and more readily accomplished in the sometimes highly charged (political?) environment which surrounds the delegation of duties in a hospital. However, this new approach is justified because of the opportunity it offers for significant improvements in the quality of health care. I believe dedicated health care professionals have that purpose uppermost in their minds. Modest administrative accommodations can be made and some liberties can be taken in implementing the proposal. In the following paragraphs is an outline of the critical features of the system theory and function so persons who seek to adapt rather than adopt will know what harm they might cause by their changes or where the proposal has some resiliency to allow alterations that will not have a material adverse effect.

The basic quality of the system is that it represents a unified approach, not the outgrowth of traditional activities but a recognition of a goal and the pursuit of it with available resources. Unification provides a logical continuum of flow from concept of a therapeutic modality in the hospital to its ultimate use in a patient and an evaluation thereafter. The total responsibility for parenteral drug administration (and even oral dosage forms, if desired) is assigned. Participants can rely on the logic of the system to reason to anything which is not clear. Active persons have identifiable functions. In some very important parts of the system, more than one discipline is assigned the same duty. This overlap is intentional. Finally, there is expertise at each point in the system. People are doing things which flow naturally from their respective education and experience backgrounds.

Here is a description of how the system operates. Purchasing specifications for standard parts of the parenterals system should be developed as the initial step of any procurement and utilization procedure. This step is important to establish baseline values for the system and to relate how its elements will function independently and with each other. Those who use the system and others with applicable expertise should participate in specification writing and approval.

The purchasing group of the hospital is the most qualified to conduct the procurement of various products. While it may seem to some people that the same group charged with the acquisition of janitorial supplies and foodstuffs may not be suitable for the purchase of drugs and large volume parenteral solutions, if specifications are written lucidly and completely, the professional purchasing agent almost invariably will do a better job than any other individual in preparing and executing the necessary contracts. These individuals have skills in negotiation, payment scheduling, delivery details and vendor guarantees which are essential to the successful completion of a procurement.

Receipt of products can be managed by any one of several techniques which suit the hospital. Records should show when material arrives and its consignment within the hospital complex. Some would suggest that lot numbers of everything purchased be kept. While the reason for this recommendation, to facilitate a search for faulty products, is commendable, the record keeping burden is immense, and the total process is questionably cost-effective.

Storage of all elements, particularly drugs and disposables, deserves care and attention. Some products must be refrigerated; others must never be cooled. Exposure to dampness, excess heat or freezing temperatures may degrade materials and render them ineffective. Even worse, the effects of a deleterious storage environment may not be apparent when the product is used, causing confusion and frustration for medical personnel and increased risk of toxicity to the patient.

Somehow, storage areas in many hospitals are next to the boiler room or power plant, in the passageway for the major steampipes, in the sub-basement where water collects or in unheated outside auxiliary buildings. In the team approach proposed here, one person must have authority, responsibility and knowledge to allocate the products to storage areas that are safe and maintained properly. This duty is properly that of a pharmacist who has additional training in handling inventories of supplies and drugs. Having a professional overview of this important function strengthens a typically weak link in the integrity of a drug-handling system and assures other members of the health care team the products they use will be of the quality intended by the manufacturer.

When the time comes to take products from storage and prepare them for use, new persons assume important roles. Staff pharmacists and technicians assisting them dominate for a period of time. They match incoming orders to available inventory (this dissertation assumes a unit dose concept for medication dispensing; modifications would be required for other systems even though the basic philosophy is retained).

Parenteral fluid units that require no admixture can be labelled appropriately and delivered to the patient care unit with little interim handling. Wherever possible, this approach should be taken to eliminate the small risk of error or contamination which accompanies manipulations in the pharmacy.

There are several products which can be purchased now that previously required admixture. These are terminally sterilized units of drugs for which there is a common dose or doses and include several different combinations of potassium chloride and either 5% dextrose or 0.9% saline solution, lidocaine, some antibiotics and even heparin in saline. There will be more of these commercially made admixtures available in the future. While the price/unit of these products may seem high at first glance, consider the significant reduction in risk to the patient deriving from the nearly zero potential for contamination and dosage calculation error. Improved quality and reduced jeopardy always increase apparent cost in the health care setting. The real benefit may be hidden and difficult to quantitate in terms of money.

When an admixture must be made at the pharmacy, if possible it should be part of a bulk preparation freeze/thaw regimen (see Chapter 6). The attributes of this approach have been described. This system should take care of most needs. In the event an unique order is received which is not likely to be required again and does not deserve integration into the overall system, the classical admixture technology should be executed, accompanied by as many checks and balances as seem reasonable.

Administration of parenteral drugs (or all drugs) should be under the immediate direction and control of a clinical pharmacist stationed in the patient care area. This emerging concept has merit. Some may see it as a further limitation on contact of the nurse with the patient at the professional level. I do not view it as such but rather feel (1) the approach assigns a responsibility for drugs to a person trained primarily for such duties, and (2) the nurse will have time to give increased patient attention for which he/she is educated. Future experiences will teach us how these two professional disciplines, pharmacist and nurse, will interact most effectively for the ultimate benefit of the patient.

It must be recognized, particularly for parenteral fluids, that the complexity of administration techniques is increasing constantly. Reference to the table of contents of this book will show the era is long past of the bottle, tube and needle approach. Very sophisticated hardware such as pumps with microprocessors and advanced types of software (catheters, new administration set configurations, etc.) are becoming the practice rather than the exception. Clinical pharmacists are being trained to select those system elements which will do no harm to drug efficacy and to administer drugs in a way the intended therapeutic purpose is achieved. More will be said on the subject later in this section. Also, the reader will find further enlightment with regard to this evolution in the portion on i.v. teams.

Blood levels (sometimes tissue levels rather than blood levels) of drugs are generally what make them work. Not all compounds remain in the blood for long periods of time. Some are metabolized rapidly by various enzymes; others bind quickly to tissue. However, many pharmaceutical preparations which are given parenterally, such as antibiotics, are beneficial only if they are given so as to maintain a detectable blood level. A study of their performance which depicts the introduction, presence and dissipation of a drug is called the *kinetics of the drug*. Recently, it has been appreciated that an understanding of a drug's kinetics can enhance the efficacy of the therapy. Too low a blood concentration usually minimizes the desired result; too high a level may induce adverse effects or even serious toxicity.

The measurement of blood levels of drugs (or of urine, bile, spinal fluid, etc.) has been facilitated by the availability of various testing kits. Presently, the laboratory in the hospital which makes the assay seems to be determined by the technology employed: nuclear medicine for radioimmunoassay, clinical chemistry for enzyme methods, immunology when an antigen–antibody (non-RIA) is being used. This disparate activity often leads to confusion and poor service. Even the most adept manager and co-ordinator cannot manipulate all the personalities in these individual estates.

The best arrangement would be for a distinct laboratory to be established in the domain of the pharmacy where these assays, regardless of technology, can be performed with suitable controls. While there may be a duplication of some equipment, the overall benefit is positive.

Along with the laboratory should be developed a true expertise in the understanding and use of various kinetic theories which characterize different drugs. All clinical pharmacists should have a working knowledge in this intellectual area so they can consult with physicians. In larger services and/or in teaching hospitals, pharmacists with advanced training in kinetics are quite useful and important, as these patient care facilities tend to receive the more critically ill who can benefit most from this advanced science.

Regardless of the brilliance with which a drug is given, there will be patients who exhibit adverse effects. It is important that everyone who sees the patient is alert to evidences for these signs and symptoms. A sensitivity to the reactions typically associated with the drugs being given is a very useful body of information for all to have. The evolution of improvements in hospital charts has not included specific places where expectations can be delineated. Generally, it is assumed that somehow people will know what is expected. With the myriad of drugs being given to individual patients, there should be a place to list *possible* adverse reactions to the specific drugs being given. The list could be on the front of the chart, updated by the clinical pharmacist as the patient drug profile changes. To avoid extemporaneous creativity and to be sure there is general agreement about the adverse effects to be listed, the Pharmacy and Therapeutics committee should approve the list to be used each time it authorizes the addition of a new drug in the hospital. Of course, it should be understood by all that the list is not the limit of their observations and that other aberrant findings can be caused by a drug. Diligence in searching out adverse effects or in recognizing early, often subtle signs must be exercised by all members of the patient care team.

The analysis of purported adverse effects is the burden of attending physicians with the assistance of clinical pharmacists. In this type of exercise knowledge of blood levels and kinetics is extremely helpful in determining what is an adverse drug effect and what is something else.

The reader might wonder by now why the changes urged above are necessary. There are many different reasons, including personnel efficiency improvements, safety factors and better drug handling. The most important reason is the changing nature of the drugs themselves. Therapeutic formulations today are more potent than ever before. They have a greater potential to produce the desired result than predecessor agents, but they also have an increased possibility of doing harm if handled incorrectly or casually. Stated in one phrase – the therapeutic index of modern drugs is smaller than previous agents.

To get the best result with least risk, special dosing sometimes is required. Additional expertise is necessary to achieve this goal. Changes proposed in both organization and responsibility are designed to provide the patient with care consistent with the evolution of these new drugs.

I.V. TEAMS

In this part of the chapter, I will describe the *raison d'etre* for infusion (i.v.) teams as part of a hospital patient care structure. Comment is provided on the 'why' and 'how' of this service which is relatively new to the hospital environment. There is a discussion of the mission of such groups and their implementation, organization, training and limits of service.

The purpose usually given for the formation of an i.v. team is that it will provide uniform service and give special attention to the initiation and maintenance of parenteral infusions. Almost with equal consistency, during the debate about whether or not to have an i.v. team, the hospital administration (or even the nursing service) will raise the question of cost effectiveness. 'Are there really sufficient problems in our institution to justify a special group of people for which there is no direct cost reimbursement?' The issue is not one to be fought on the balance sheet, for one major adverse incident more than consumes the time and talent of personnel which could have been allocated to i.v. team activities. The real question is whether such a service can be activated and sustained professionally in order for it to yield patient benefits and efficiencies for which it is designed. If the team members do nothing more than start intravenous infusions so other nurses and house physicians are relieved to do whatever (usually nothing definitive or identifiable), an i.v. team is an unnecessary luxury. When the team fulfills its mission and adds to the quality and efficiency of care and comfort of the patient, its existence is justified, and another major improvement is added to the hospital environment.

Initial personnel for an i.v. team usually are recruited from nurses who are working in the hospital already. The team leader is a person who can see the program in full bloom (or destroy the concept completely for many years to come at the institution). He/she should have leadership qualities, some administrative expertise, and above all a willingness, even an anxiety, to participate in the daily duties of the team and to be expert in team patient care functions. The remainder of the team personnel should want something more than better hours and less routine. Escapists from floor nursing rarely serve a long tenure on an i.v. team and contribute little to its overall effectiveness. Although it seems disloyal, sometimes it is better to find team personnel, particularly in the beginning, on the 'outside' so they come unencumbered with endogenous traditions and prejudices. Very often membership is restricted to nurses, but I believe all i.v. teams would be enhanced in their function if they included the active participation of a pharmacist. As will be seen, many team functions have a pharmacy flavor. An equally valuable feature is an interested physician consultant and/or advisor. Both the external politics and the internal workings of the team can be helped considerably by such persons.

The first action in implementing an i.v. team is to define its responsibilities. A full menu would include the following:

(1) Start all routine intravenous infusions and maintain the vein access as long as an order remains in force to do so. This duty should be seen as including catheters that are in place for emergency use (such as coronary care unit patients) but not serving

regularly as a conduit for fluid. These devices have equal potential for complications as do working catheters.

(2) Maintain and be knowledgeable about intra-arterial lines, including dressing changes and the routine care thereof.

(3) If permitted by the medical staff (rarely), insert central venous
catheters. Even if not inserted by team members, these catheters
should be managed by the team to the exclusion of other hospital
personnel.

(4) Start blood transfusions and infusion of other blood products,
particularly those which depend for their safety on proper patient/
unit identification.

(5) Participate in the selection of all vascular access disposables
(except Swan Ganz and cardiac catheters); establish thoughtful
protocols for their use and provide service for them.

Things which the team and/or its leader *should not do* are:

(1) Become involved in the purchasing policies of the hospital. Team
advice should be at the professional level exclusively.

(2) Restrict their patient care participation to infusions only, even
though it is clear in certain situations their assistance is needed
and wanted ('it's not my job').

(3) Take command in an emergency circumstance because they know
some pharmacology (unless they are designated to so).

Conceivably, an adept i.v. team can also include in its purview some
role in the use of infusion control permanent equipment such as pumps.
Team members should have sufficiently extensive knowledge to provide
meaningful assistance and training in this area to general duty nurses. I
believe a better result will be forthcoming when i.v. team personnel are
involved intimately in such apparatus. The biomedical engineer or
maintenance department seem hardly the place for handling pumps
other than to repair them and check their function.

After personnel the next serious issue is training. Initially i.v. team
members should have the benefit of lectures in the anatomy and physiology of the cardiovascular system. Pressures found normally in different
parts of the circulation should be well known. Of course, a working
knowledge of the superficial vein structure, especially the related muscle
and bone landmarks, is essential to the successful insertion of vein access
devices, needles or catheters, when adequate filling does not delineate
the vessel. There is hardly a more impressive clinical feat than to
penetrate an unseen vein deftly and with proper technique and style on

61

the first attempt. To obtain this teaching, the services of the hospital anesthesia department can be solicited. An alternate may be an advanced graduate student in human anatomy from a nearby medical school. Some pathology should also be included in the education. Team people should understand phlebitis, suppuration, abscess, thrombosis, foreign body reaction, embolus and bacteremia. Only elemental details are necessary, but without them team members will not have a perception of the various disease processes they encounter.

A truly important element in the training curriculum is that of routines to be used in establishing patient identity, particularly if the team is to be involved in blood products administration. An absolute protocol must be adopted from existing practice or created *de novo* with the assistance and consent of appropriate medical staff committees. It must be understood by all, and followed without exception. Permissible shortcuts in emergencies should be anticipated in the protocol, not created as the need arises in a crisis situation. The protocol, often called a standard operating procedure (SOP), should be published as part of the hospital rules.

A sometimes overlooked part of the training program is the plan for orientation of new team members subsequent to the first group. Commonly, there are only one or two replacements brought in at a time, and mounting a full teaching schedule is unrealistic logistically. Sadly, new people get their training by apprenticeship in many instances, a wholly inadequate substitute for the real thing. As more people on the team take the primary course from others, the total knowledge base diminishes and ultimately disintegrates completely. I can make no definitive recommendation to solve this problem but only note its existence. Perhaps some enterprising commercial organization will step into the void.

Another cause of poor training occurs in the rush to replace a team member who has resigned unexpectedly or become ill. A new person is recruited hurriedly, without training, and thrust into the work shift of the departed with the expectation there will be time later for the niceties. But alas, the time never comes, and another person has joined the outfit truly unfit for duty. For this problem I do have a suggestion. Have the next member picked, trained and ready to go, waiting for the opportunity on the reserve roster. In this way training can be done at a leisurely pace. The thrill of anticipating the new assignment also adds to the enthusiasm of the individual.

Last to be mentioned in this section on implementation, but not least important, is the design and pursuit of a monitoring system – a quality control activity. No team should be without one, but many are. A good monitor system is much more than a tabulation of traffic: how many starts, how many patients, how much supplies, etc. The team should have a time related report, monthly is a good frequency, on infiltrations, incidence of phlebitis, sepsis, equipment failure, disposable malfunction and faults and all related matters. To do this job well cards should be made out for all patients seen, with identifying information that will permit a trace to the full hospital record if necessary. On the card there should appear an outline of the vascular anatomy to depict the location of each i.v. started by the team. Columns of information should include the date and hour, device used, name of team member providing the service and space for observations as to outcome with a check mark suitable for routine endpoints (order discontinued, etc.) or narrative for other events. Another card should be completed when an adverse incident occurs. This record should be given to the member of the team assigned to quality control monitoring, a duty which can be rotated among personnel for 3 month periods. It is the responsibility of this person to organize the agenda for a monthly morbidity conference which all team personnel attend, especially the physician consultant/adviser and pharmacist. Health care professionals learn from mistakes, and strong i.v. team members seek to benefit from their miscues and errors. If an increase in the incidence of phlebitis is seen by relating new data to historical information, an investigation should be initiated for possible causes. The individual patient cards serve handsomely when this action is necessary. Interaction with other hospital services such as infection control is also important.

Continuing education has become a real tour de force in medicine with nearly every accreditation, licensing and regulating agency demanding some evidence for its existence. Team personnel have a special mission in patient care, and they should recognize the opportunities afforded by continuing education. This statement is not meant to be interpreted as a justification for attending out of town conventions. Good teams have regular, internal education activities at which members prepare presentations for others or outside experts present their thoughts on new equipment or techniques. When done in house, there are benefits to the teacher as well as the taught. There is nothing more challenging than an assignment to prepare a teaching presentation for one's peers.

At some point during the decision process to have an i.v. team, the question arises about which major hospital function will have the group – where it will report. Perhaps because most personnel are nurses, the choice usually favors the nursing service. However, I suggest an alternate which hopefully is interesting and even viable in several places. I believe the pharmacy is a good home for the i.v. team. Parenteral fluids more and more are vehicles for drugs, and drugs involve the pharmacy. With the advent of central admixture and the general management of parenteral fluids by the pharmacy, the i.v. team seems to fit naturally in that domain. Especially in hospitals where clinical pharmacy has established a strong foothold, this marriage is one of convenience and mutual benefit. The combination can make an excellent total medication delivery unit.

One innovative group has reported their i.v. team nurses on a single occasion and under supervision make a few admixtures. The theory is that by making some of the product to be given, the i.v. team nurse learns more about his/her business and that of others to which they relate. Team members understand the problems of admixture and what to look for to identify them properly.

Within the total organizational structure of the patient care staff of the hospital, the i.v. team leader should be invited to serve (*ex officio* if not officially) on the nutrition committee and the infection committee. The relationship to each is obvious.

An i.v. team serves several purposes. It provides professional attention for a frequent and sometimes complex kind of medical care. At least one third of all patients receive an infusion during their hospital stay; many sources say this value can reach 75% of patients, depending upon which medical specialties dominate the inpatient population. The care is rendered efficiently with attention to standards that make treatment safe and effective. Quality control for infusions can be established and sustained. With records to serve as a base, methods improvement can be implemented. Complex apparatus and ever changing technology are handled better by a specialist compared to a generalist. There is likely to be a concurrent reduction of risk for adverse reactions such as infection, drug and blood incompatibilities and apparatus malfunction due to abuse or misuse. Above all, better patient care can result from the participation of an i.v. team in the hospital services.

SUMMARY

The infusion service is a complex of interacting functions which must integrate well to serve the hospital environment successfully. An organization quite different from that frequently seen has been proposed (and justified?). The pharmacist is the health care professional who should have the primary responsibility in the hospital.

I.v. team structure and function should emphasize training and monitoring of results. A professional attitude must pervade the group. The team should be responsible to the pharmacist.

6
Admixtures

The purposes of this chapter are (1) to describe the dominant admixture technologies now in use, (2) to picture a typical organization for a pharmacy operated central admixture program, (3) to present the advantages and disadvantages of nurse prepared and pharmacy prepared admixtures, and (4) to offer a recently developed alternative which embodies some new concepts for preparing, testing and storing admixtures.

A rather strict definition of admixture was published by a national group in 1975 – 'a large volume parenteral to which one or more additional drug products have been added in the hospital'. I think the definition is unduly restrictive because (1) the same authority states a large volume parenteral is a sterile solution of 100 ml or more and (2) the location of preparation is limited to the hospital. A preferred definition, more in keeping with the current times, would be 'a solution intended for intravascular administration by other than rapid injection which has been prepared in part by the addition of ingredients after terminal sterilization of one or more of the components *or* the container'. The difference between these definitions is intended to recognize the emerging dominance of 50 ml piggyback containers and the increasing frequency of orders for parenteral nutrition solution, usually mixed into an empty container, which may be considered the ultimate in admixtures as will be explained in Chapter 13.

There are five major types of admixtures: (1) Large volume, (2) piggyback, (3) irrigating solutions, (4) parenteral nutrition, and (5) drugs. Until recently, addition of the potassium ion to dextrose or saline in 500 or 1000 ml containers was the most common admixture ordered and prepared. Because potassium containing solutions are inherently heat and time stable, several commercial firms have made them available as a pre-mixed, terminally sterilized product. Such solutions should be chosen over any pharmacy or nurse made solution because they have the protection of terminal sterilization. Solutions containing lidocaine or heparin, commonly employed in emergency rooms and coronary care units, also can be purchased and obviate the need for admixture.

The 'piggyback' solution is a container usually of smaller volume than the primary infusion; it is connected from time to time during a 24 hour period to the main fluid delivery system in order to provide a therapeutic agent on an intermittent basis. The most common 'piggyback' is an antibiotic, but there are many others (cimetidine, etc.). Sometimes physicians want to use an irrigating solution containing a therapeutic agent. These must be prepared as an admixture as they are rarely available commercially. Although irrigating solutions are applied commonly to external body surfaces, their use in body cavities (for instance, the urinary bladder) and the possibility of systemic absorption in some instances mandates that admixtures used in this manner be prepared and treated with essentially the same respect as those for intravascular use. Irrigating solution containers have several different closure systems, so special techniques for making and protecting the admixture are required. In my opinion none are entirely suitable, and irrigating solution admixtures should be approached with great caution.

Parenteral nutrition mixtures need little explanation other than mention of the name. A separate chapter has been written on this subject (Chapter 13) where preparation of a parenteral nutrition admixture is presented.

Drug admixtures are increasingly popular with the advent of extended infusion antitumor chemotherapy and the commercial availability of frozen admixtures of antibiotics and other therapeutic agents.

Until relatively recently all admixtures were made in patient care areas by the professional nursing staff. At least 50% of hospitals continue to function in this way. Several texts have been written on the subject. If the hospital has a nurse prepared admixture policy, it should have a uniform policy and procedure for nurse guidance which can be presented to and studied by new employees and reviewed during in service sessions. A senior person in the nursing service should have the responsibility for being cognizant of the changing picture in admixtures, such as the announcement of any incompatibilities or the availability of new equipment. When a new device is introduced into hospital practice, no effort should be spared to make certain that all personnel are familiar with it and practiced in its use.

If there is to be no central admixture service, every nursing station must have a space specifically designated to make admixtures. It should remain sacrosanct, well equipped, and protected from abuses such as the storage of non-admixture materials, patient specimens and other clutter. Its sink should not be used to wash coffee cups, and its waste container must be reserved only for the excesses of admixture. To the extent possible the admixture area at each nursing station throughout the hospital should have the same configuration. This nicety makes teaching more effective and provides a stronger basis for uniform procedures, quality monitoring, and a means to assess the benefits and adversities of contemplated changes in standard procedures.

The nurse prepares an admixture usually from a vial of drug already in a liquid form or by means of reconstituting a lyophilized (freeze-dried) product. For the latter a reconstitution device is available, designed for use with plastic containers. (Figure 6.1) It facilitates sterile transfer by

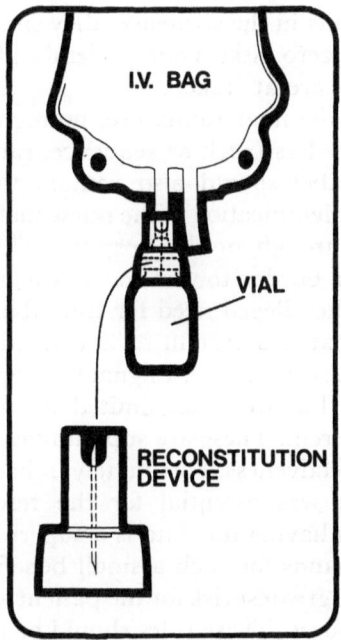

Figure 6.1 A reconstitution device which is actually a double end needle that is protected by a hood to prevent touch contamination

limiting the access of fingers to the exposed surfaces of the diluent containing bag and the drug containing vial. Because there is no means of metering the quantity of diluent, the reconstitution device is limited to dosage containers intended for transfer of the entire vial content. Multiple doses from the same vial are precluded.

A more common technique for transferring a drug to a final container is to use a syringe and needle. The liquid form of a drug concentrate, initial or reconstituted, is removed from the original vial in the calculated quantity and injected into the parenteral container. If several units of the same kind are to be made, the temptation to load the syringe for all of them at one time should be avoided, particularly for vacuum packed glass containers. It is not possible to maintain adequate accuracy in consecutive transfers. Each maneuver should be performed individually. Failure to do so is a potential source of serial contamination of units.

Each large volume parenteral system has unique attributes for the sterility of the surfaces involved with admixture. Likewise, small vials of concentrated drugs have closure systems of several types. You must be certain of the manufacturer's directions in the use of these units. If a surface is contaminated accidentally, or even if there is the slightest suspicion of such abuse, full decontamination treatment must precede the next step in admixture manipulation. If there is a doubt about previously prepared units in the sequence, they should be discarded and made again. Work to zero risk! Your patient's life and possibly your professional reputation are at stake.

A label is affixed to the final admixture, noting the patient who is to receive it and special orders (such as sequence, rate, etc.) governing its administration. The label should also contain the date and time of preparation and some identification of the nurse making it. Labels should be constant in form throughout the hospital. They should not be so complex as to become a burden to write or meaningless because they are illegible. Justified by the alleged need for traceability, in the past some authorities have advocated a system of documentation that is rivaled only by the federal bureaucracy. Designated suggested spaces on the format have included, but were not limited to, the lot number of all materials contained therein. These are superfluities which seem interesting but have no cost effectiveness. Fortunately, it has been a rare instance that such information was essential for the resolution of a clinical problem. In such cases having the data is a superb discovery. However, burdening many thousands for such a small benefit is not reasonable.

Contamination is the greatest risk for the patient and touch contamination is the dominant source. These rules should be followed to avoid this fault:

(1) Wash your hands. Do not prepare admixtures if you have open sores on your hands.

(2) Know the intricacies of the containers, appliances and tubing you will be using. There are several different mechanical systems; each requires unique manipulations to be worked properly. Do not use a system with which you have no practice or for which you are not trained. The likelihood is substantial for inadvertent abuse which may escape unnoticed.

(3) Clean the area in which you will be making the admixtures

68

immediately before you work on it. Do not trust cleaning to others. Be fastidious.

(4) Follow a constant pattern of work, one of your own innovation or another you may have learned. Be deliberate and systematic. Do the same things in the same way each time. Do not tolerate an interruption during the process of admixture preparation. Be away from the main flow of traffic.

(5) Label everything clearly and completely, including source components. Others may be involved in administering or monitoring your work product. They should know who made it and when, for whom it is intended, and how it is to be given. If you do not know, don't make the admixture.

There has been a long tradition in nursing practice to 'give what you make'. The ostensible purpose was to avoid errors in giving and receiving instructions or transferring responsibility at meal breaks and shift changes. The complexities of nursing station routine and the patterns of patient care organization make this directive increasingly difficult to prosecute. While its advantage is obvious and the more subtle feature of limiting the burden of a mistake to a single person who can be identified later is theoretically attractive, placing blame for an unhappy incident hardly seems a sound motivation for sustaining inefficiencies. The practice of 'give what you make' is becoming an anachronism in many hospitals.

The emerging technology for parenteral admixtures is control in the central pharmacy of the hospital. There are many reasons for this change, some very real and others rather meaningless from the patient's viewpoint. Among the latter is the often expressed statement that control of admixtures improves the professional standing of the pharmacist in the health care structure. Another reason is that it is unfair 'to literally dump their (pharmacists) responsibilities on the nursing supervisor after 5 p.m. and on weekends'.

Fortunately, these concepts are supervened by several persuasive ideas which merit the attention of all persons interested in admixture. Among them are the instructive findings of Thur and colleagues who showed that several errors occurred during a nurse staffed admixture system. For instance, they found 21 medication errors in 100 parenteral admixtures prepared by nurses. There were 271 interruptions of the nurses while they were preparing the 100 admixtures. On 15 occasions it appeared to the investigators that the nurse should have sought additional information before initiating or completing the admixture. There were several technique errors noted. The study did not include a bacterial surveillance component so it is not possible to know how many of these faults resulted in contamination of the admixture.

The central admixture program, by definition, is geographically distant from the sites of patient care. This fact, and recognition that another team is involved, mandates a well orchestrated system of communication, response and verification. There is no room for a constant flow of complaints and accusations intended to place the burden of a missed medication; only the patient suffers.

CENTRAL ADMIXTURE

Preparation of drug admixtures at a central location, almost always the hospital pharmacy, is a present day reality in an increasing percentage of hospitals in the United States. In the United Kingdom such a program has not emerged as fully. There are several excellent reasons for assigning admixture responsibility to the pharmacy. Here are the more obvious:

(1) The complexities of admixture preparation require special training for proper understanding and implementation. A nurses' curriculum or in service education program does not address these matters effectively.

(2) Allocation of proper space in each patient care area for preparation of admixtures (where nothing else occurs) is not feasible, given the overcrowding that exists already. The cost of such space in new construction is prohibitive. Therefore, any location in a nurses station is shared with other functions. The traffic patterns in such areas develop hostile environments for safe preparation of admixtures.

(3) When a nurse prepares admixtures, a costly and sometimes critically short talent is being used to the exclusion of activities for which it is better suited. The system has neither a favorable cost effectiveness nor an attractive risk benefit.

(4) No quality control system is possible. If a consistent technique error is made which endangers patients, there is no way to detect it. These errors include, but are not limited to, bacterial contamination, dosage miscalculation and a mixture of physical/chemical drug incompatibilities.

In spite of the above some hospitals simply cannot accommodate a central admixture program. In general these would be institutions having fewer than 200 beds where personnel arrangements preclude accomplishment of the work in the pharmacy. Later in this chapter I will describe a new technique which can resolve this difficulty. For very large hospitals where the geography appears to preclude efficient admixture preparation centrally, the same new approach will work nicely.

For this part of the discussion it will be presumed the location of admixture preparation is the hospital pharmacy, and the ultimate individual responsible for the function is the hospital pharmacy director. The important issue is to understand principles underlying central admixture so they form the foundation of the organization and function of the service. The most important single factor is *'Quality and safety are built into the product'*. Wherever the location of the admixture preparation area, a sign with these words should be placed prominently on each of the nearby walls. Not a piece of paper with words typed on it and hung with some tape. Instead, a professionally lettered, framed placard (which shows that you mean business). Remember, quality cannot be *tested into* the product. The hospital pharmacist sets the tone. Every word and action should exude these concepts. No compromises, no shortcuts and no accommodations.

When an admixture is prepared from products supplied by a commercial source, the manufacturer's warranty of safety and effectiveness may be abrogated considerably, and the pharmacy assumes at least some of the burden previously carried by the vendor. This statement is not a legal opinion. It is a conclusion based on the fact that vendor sourced product is being manipulated by other than the vendor, possibly in a manner not anticipated by the seller in the physical or chemical design.

Under ideal circumstances the preparation of admixtures has the appearance of a quasi-production setting. Fullest advantage should be taken of automated equipment to the extent justified by volume, thereby eliminating the chance for human error. Admittedly, devices can function improperly, creating an immense number of mistakes. The trade-offs between human and machine error have been studied many times, and machines win. (Today it is called robotics.) They can be monitored and analyzed more conveniently and effectively. Admixture orders should be grouped, an arrangement facilitated by having good communication with patient care areas. Also necessary is some willingness to risk preparation of units in anticipation of use during the day. The hospital administration should understand there may be a small waste factor derived from units that are not ordered within 24 hours of preparation. Good record keeping will minimize the cost of these units overall. Admixtures with very costly components probably should not be included in such a pre-order prediction mechanism.

An interesting economic advantage for the volume production approach can be the use of multi dose source drug units which reduce the cost per dose significantly. All of these factors add up to the need for careful and thoughtful monitoring of this pharmacy service by a professional person who is devoted to its effective operation.

When admixture orders are received in the pharmacy, a professional pharmacist with experience and an inquisitive mind should review each one for established physical and chemical compatibility of the components and reasonableness of the dose. This examination should have a positive connotation. The order should be processed only if the reviewer knows it can be made and administered safely instead of stopping the order only if the pharmacist is sure something is wrong. Textbook and literature consultation, professional service groups in vendor organizations, and colleagues at pharmacy schools should be consulted if there is doubt. Also, the ordering physician should be contacted to discuss the situation. Almost everyone will be grateful for the call, even when there are nearly no facts to support a real concern but only a missing confirmation of safety and effectiveness. Those who are ungrateful can be tolerated with the understanding there are always an aberrant few. Their wrath is easily sustainable in the knowledge the right thing was done.

Presuming a pharmacy admixture operation of reasonable size, orders can be grouped and prepared by technicians. This personnel level has been an important addition to pharmacy practice and should be included wherever possible to have a well balanced work force. Unfortunately, as yet no career path has emerged for these employees so there is a higher than usual turnover and in some a lack of motivation. Efforts should be made to correct this defect in personnel administration.

The work of a technician is to prepare the admixture, using data supplied by the pharmacist or schedules which are routine in the facility. Even complex admixtures can be handled by technicians when there is proper professional pharmacy supervision.

Technician training has become a favorite subject for several authors in recent years. Each has a new or different twist, but they all add up to the same thing. You must have absolute faith and trust in the talent of technicians before releasing them for production activities. There is no monitoring system that can detect every technician induced fault. The philosophy for the final approval of a technician by a pharmacist should be 'I know they can perform better than me' versus 'I don't see anything wrong so probably they are okay'.

The basic education of a technician candidate should be at the high school completion level. They should possess a better than average facility with mathematics. During the interview process they should impress everyone with evidences of personal habits of cleanliness and good grooming. Technician candidates should exemplify a nascent sense of professional esteem, and be able to learn an appreciation for the pivotal role of the pharmacy in patient care as well as the technical details of the science to which they will be exposed.

Work of the technician must be verified by the supervising pharmacist, meaning there are sufficient evidences of what was done to create an audit trail that can reconstruct the work which was performed. The finished products and some pieces of paper to be signed for release are not enough. Empty vials and units of diluent, calculations which show the quantity of starting material and the estimates of end product, records which include lot numbers and even labels of raw materials where feasible, and a completed procedure check list should be presented to the supervisor. Where it is not possible to do all these things, a pre-action check of materials and equipment set up to do the work should be made by the pharmacist supervisor.

I believe in signatures which indicate a function has been performed or a check has been made. Putting a signature on the line adds a dimension to the total perception of responsibility for both the technician and pharmacist (and everyone else for that matter). Everything related to a preparation activity should be dated and signed, not to fix blame if a mistake occurs (because it will) but to facilitate the search process, isolate the problem, minimize its impact, and learn how to avoid it.

An admixture should be labelled clearly with the information necessary for its proper use. Data should include at least the name of the patient for whom the order is intended, the patient's hospital location and hospital number, the usual details about content of the container, the intended method of administration, the date of preparation and the date and hour of expiration (since it is to be sent from a distant source versus the nurse prepared admixture), and the date and hour of intended use if it is reasonable to provide such information in accordance with physician's orders. This array of numbers may appear to be useless in part, but an item by item examination will show the value of each. Of course, signature initials (not typed) of the preparing technician and the releasing pharmacist must be on the label also.

Admixtures are sent to patient areas as soon as they are released in accordance with a medication order. They should not be stored in any floor refrigerator which happens to be convenient. Just because an admixture container looks like it is impervious to a hostile environment does not mean it can be subject to constant challenge. Admixtures should have a specific, unique, recognized location from which they can be picked up and taken to the bedside. The nurse should verify the content stated on the label is consistent with the physician's order. Then the nurse should also initial the label, signifying participation in the process. Hospital rules for administration should be written and followed explicitly. The patient must be identified by name, number and location. If any of the facts are at variance with the admixture label, consultation with the pharmacy should ensue immediately. It is the responsibility of the nurse to administer the admixture in accordance with the label. If it differs from the physician's order, a resolution must be reached. If an untoward problem occurs during the use of the admixture, or even shortly thereafter and possibly related to it, the pharmacy should be notified by the nurse. All but the most simple and obvious situations should be explored jointly with the physician and/or house staff involved.

The most important point has been saved until last in this section. Until now I have made only perfunctory mention of quality control in admixture preparation. During the past 5 years there has been a plethora of papers on the subject, most describing a particular technique or statistical approach with accompanying claims for superiority because of a special feature(s). Statesmen in the pharmacy profession have written editorials for every available journal on the subject. Where there are no data, there are always philosophies. Quality control is 'in'.

The Joint Commission on Accreditation of Hospitals (USA) has made pharmacy quality control a leading feature in its overall quality monitoring undertaking in hospitals. Among the various aspects of inpatient care, the pharmacy and the clinical laboratory offer products which are relatively easy to monitor and evaluate. Thus, these areas have become early targets for inquiry and inspection by Joint Commission representatives.

In preparing this text, it was necessary to decide how to handle the subject of quality control; how much detail to present, and how firm to stand behind a single approach to the exclusion of others. After studying much of what was available, I decided that there were several facts which merited communication to the reader:

(1) Not everything published is correct in general; sometimes procedures are based on statistical principles that are not proper for the issues being treated.

(2) Not everything published is correct for a particular environment; sometimes features in the statistics (although technically correct) do not fit the intended application.

(3) Not everything published works as advertised; for instance in the presentation of complex statistical equations and sequences, a printing error can go unrecognized by those who seek to apply mechanically what they have learned (but not understood) from the paper.

(4) Essentially everything focuses upon microbial quality, the absence of bacterial contamination. Nearly nothing is said about potency errors in prepared units.

The most difficult problems in devising a proper quality control system for admixture preparation are these:

(1) Whatever method is selected will have its impact retrospectively; because cultures usually take at least 24 hours to grow and

74

indicate a fault, all of the product being studied is used when a potential problem is detected. Even more interesting (and fortunate) is that the consequence of infusing a faulty admixture often is not manifest by the patient. Confidence in the quality control system, not the process being studied, is undermined because it may appear to be generating false positives.

(2) Quality control of admixtures is an issue of sampling strategy in which it is admitted that a small level of contaminated, poor quality units may be released undetected. How is the acceptable level of dangerous product selected, knowing that any single one may cause serious harm you are sworn to avoid as a member of the health care profession?

(3) A good job of quality control costs money, and except for regulatory or JCAH demands, it is an ethereal concept which may be hard to sell to a cost conscious administration. In any cost cutting program quality control often is the first victim. Until some adverse event of significance, the value of quality control may be unrecognized because the real risks are hard to appreciate.

(4) Given a well organized admixture service, process aberrations, often of a consistent or systematic type, will be found. Individual problems may go undetected, or, if identified, will not be verified because the companion units may not exhibit the same quality fault.

Upon reading this list of challenges, one might wonder why a reasonable person would try to provide a quality control feature in central admixture technology. To be sure, the best protection of quality is intelligent formulation of a preparation process and strict, undeviating adherence to it ('Quality and safety are built into the product'). The purposes of monitoring procedures are to find unsuspected deterioration in the process (filtration faults, equipment failures), to identify the introduction of any variables which challenge the basis on which the system was built (a careless technician, non-sterile raw materials), to locate difficulties which arise from incorrect presumptions about ancillary operating systems which are in the purview of persons beyond the pharmacy and about which the pharmacy is unlikely to be notified (house compressed air or vacuum systems not within acceptable performance limits), and to isolate outside the pharmacy (by providing demonstrable evidence to the contrary) patient care problems that might be attributed erroneously to admixture preparation, thus allowing the real source of danger to be identified rather than go uncorrected.

Since our first acquaintance I have had considerable respect for my colleague, Dr Roy Sanford, who became interested in these and related issues while serving on an expert panel for quality control. He has made a thoughtful study of the problem and devised an admixture sampling system which has broad applicability. Dr Sanford has been kind enough to provide his essay on the subject for the use of readers of this book; it is printed in the appendix. The Sanford approach has been criticized because it is too complex or too costly or too extreme. In doing so people are saying they do not understand, or they do not want so much control (or quality?). I commend Dr Sanford's work to readers in the pharmacy profession and to their consultants, and ask them to undertake a critical examination of its content. Many will find, I am sure, it has attractive features which can be applied in whole or part to individual circumstances.

Whatever system is selected, it must be understood thoroughly by the hospital pharmacist, professional pharmacy colleagues, and at least the chairman of the Pharmacy and Therapeutics Committee of the Medical Staff. These people should know what quality control is doing.

Apart from the statistical issues and sampling problems is the question of how well the detection mechanism works. What is the resolving power of the method selected to control quality? How bad must be the blunder before it can be detected by testing? How many times does the test produce a false indication of contamination, an indication of unacceptable quality when the unit was perfectly fine? By the time the conscientious pharmacist has devised a satisfactory sampling program, it is little wonder that there remains almost no appetite for evaluating and then monitoring the test itself, but to do so is a necessary component of overall quality control.

A recent paper exemplifies the problem. It showed that manipulative contamination of test units was high enough to obscure any identification of true contamination. The authors concluded that adventitious contamination (false positives) was a 'component of, and possibly a dominant factor in, the contamination rates detected by hospital sterility tests'. This circumstance is not acceptable for the proper function of quality control. The incidence of false positives (background noise) must be sufficiently low so when a positive unit is signaled in the test system, it can be pursued with a reasonable expectation that a true fault has been detected. Without such confidence the whole operation tumbles like a house of cards. (You remember – 'crying wolf'.) Making the situation more difficult is the fact that organisms expected in true contamination, hand bacteria, often are the same genus and species found in false positives. It is a question of where the contaminant enters, during preparation of the admixture (a true positive) or during testing (a false positive). Manufacturers have a much easier situation. Most authorities are willing to classify all but Gram-negative bacilli as adventitious organisms in a test system for terminally sterilized parenteral fluid.

Another evaluation of the micro-organism test is its sensitivity. The pharmacist must know the smallest number of bacterial organisms that will develop a true positive. If the test remains negative when several bacteria are present, it is hardly a test worth performing. It would give a false sense of security. For instance, a comparison of two recovery methods was reported; 72% of challenges with 15–27 spores each produced positive results in one technique, and approximately 20% of samples with 1–10 cells were identified by another technique. The remainder were false negatives (missed). I question the adequacy of either method for maintaining a quality monitor on an admixture system. A statistician providing the design for quality control must be aware of desired and actual test performance levels and accommodate the total procedure for them. These facts give support to the contention that no book formulae can be used directly. Adaptation by experienced, expert personnel is most important.

FREEZE/MICROWAVE THAW TECHNOLOGY

It can be seen easily that central admixture as practiced now is a fertile area for innovation. I have been fortunate to work with several colleagues and acquaintances in the development of a technology that appears to address most of the problem areas. The basic concept came from admiration of some very intelligent work by Dinel and associates which demonstrated the durability of several different antibiotic admixtures in plastic containers during periods of freezing. Dinel applied this concept in a fashion that allowed for the prospective preparation of many units of the same admixture at a single time followed by frozen storage until use. Thawing was done at room temperature. It was this aspect that proved the undoing of the Dinel approach on a practical basis. Thawing at 20–25 °C required 2–8 hours, depending on the size of the unit, and it became necessary for the hospital pharmacy to predict use because prospective thawing time from receipt of an order was longer than could be tolerated. Still several pharmacies applied the principle to high volume admixtures where daily use could be predicted to some extent, making up any shortages with immediate preparations.

A few years later I received a personal communication from Henry Jarocha, RPh of the Strong Memorial Hospital, University of Rochester, who mentioned the possibility of microwave energy thawing to dissipate the primary objection to freezing admixtures routinely. There followed much work, done mostly by Dr Clifford Holmes whom I had come to know and respect during his formal education at the University of Manchester, England. Working in the laboratory of Drs Ruth Kundsin and Carl Walter of the Harvard Medical School, Holmes has shown in

77

some landmark publications that nearly all antibiotics in common use today sustain freezing and microwave thawing without alteration in antibacterial potency. My colleagues Holmes, Kundsin, Walter and I were joined by Messrs Kerkhof and Cantwell in the development of proof that parenteral nutrition admixtures of crystalline amino acids and dextrose similarly can be frozen, stored and microwave thawed.

Given that the technology has been demonstrated convincingly, a discussion of the application of freeze/microwave thaw is presented for the purpose of reader orientation. To obtain a detailed view, the original papers on the subject should be consulted.

The basic concept is that nearly all admixtures of common interest can be prepared in quantities that take advantage of efficiencies and safety inherent in the use of automated equipment. Sometimes certain price advantages ensue when volume purchases of raw materials are made. Manufacturing batches are frozen immediately, and quality control becomes a prospective activity while the batch remains in unreleased control of the pharmacy until all requirements have been met. Thereupon, release to useable inventory is made.

When orders are received, admixtures are taken from released stock, placed in a microwave thawing unit of special design, and returned to the liquid state. Labelling is completed following the rules noted earlier in this chapter, and the admixtures are ready for delivery to the nursing station. If a need occurs during hours in which the pharmacy is closed, authorized and trained nursing service personnel withdraw admixtures from frozen storage and thaw them in the microwave apparatus. Thus, central admixture does not mandate 24 hour, 7 day pharmacy hours.

Several pages ago I mentioned the reality that hospitals of smaller size (less than 200 beds) might have difficulty in implementing a central admixture program. The frozen storage concept is suited ideally to a regionalized hospital pharmacy service. Larger facilities can prepare admixtures which are transported frozen after release for adequate storage at the satellite hospital site. Another option is commercial preparation when an admixture is needed; the thawing process is managed by the nurse or pharmacist on location. There are many service and economy advantages in such a system.

Quality control in the freeze–thaw procedure is a matter entirely apart from the problems seen with routine central admixture. It is more traditional because it is prospective and accommodates controls on product not otherwise possible.

SUMMARY

Central admixture is being installed in hospitals with increasing frequency as its advantages are recognized by administrators, pharmacists and nurses. The shortcomings of nurse prepared admixtures are very real and meaningful to patients. As the kinetics of drugs are understood more fully and technologies for flow control improve, agents having a therapeutic ratio indicating smaller margins of safety will be administered. Errors in preparation or the assessment of compatibility with other drugs or delivery vehicles may have substantial consequences for the patient. A controlled, well managed system of preparation for admixtures is necessary to accommodate the constantly improving techniques of drug selection and delivery. The professional pharmacist is most suited among all health care personnel to provide this service, including quality control, so that the medical and nursing staffs can have full confidence in the products they order and administer.

A new freeze/microwave thaw technique for storage, prospective quality control, release to an active inventory and final use offers advantages, particularly where existing systems are weak. This technology can bring central admixture advantages without prohibitive costs and manpower demands to many hospitals with an insufficient patient population and staff to support a full central admixture program. The time is approaching when admixture preparation under supervision of the pharmacy will be standard in hospital operation.

Bibliography

1. Department of Health and Social Security – (UK). (1976). Addition of drugs to intravenous infusion fluids. *Health Circular*, **HC(76),** 9 March
2. Brier, K. L., Latiolais, C. J., Schneider, P. J. *et. al.* (1981). Effect of laminar air flow and clean room dress on contamination rates of intravenous admixtures. *Am. J. Hosp. Pharm.*, **38,** 1144
3. Bernick, J. J., Brown, D. G. and Bell, J. E. (1979). Adventitious contamination of intravenous admixtures during sterility testing. *Am. J. Hosp. Pharm.*, **36,** 1493
4. Green, B. L. and Litsky, W. (1979). Evaluation of a closed system for sterility testing of parenterals. *Pharmaceut. Technol.*, 72
5. Thur, M. P., Miller, W. A. and Latiolais, C. J. (1972). Medication errors in a nurse controlled parenteral admixture program. *Am. J. Hosp. Pharm.*, **29,** 298
6. Stolar, M. H. (1979). National survey of hospital pharmaceutical services – 1978. *Am. J. Hosp. Pharm.*, **36,** 316
7. Plouffe, J. F., Brown, D. G., Silva, J. *et al.* (1977). Nosocomial outbreak of *candida parapsilosis fungemia* related to intravenous infusions. *Arch. Int. Med.*, **137,** 1686
8. Zellmer, W. A. (1978). Quality control in admixture services. *Am. J. Hosp. Pharm.*, **35,** 527
9. Teixeira, C. A., Kendall, R. W. and Dinel, B. A. (1973). A centralized mini-bag admixture service. *Can. J. Hosp. Pharm.*, p. 103
10. Jarocha, H. (1977). Microbiological quality control in a pharmacy. *Hosp. Pharm.*, **12,** 575
11. Stolar, M. H. (1979). Assuring the quality of intravenous admixture programs. *Am. J. Hosp. Pharm.*, **36,** 605
12. Rycroft, J. A. and Moon, D. (1975). An 'in-production' method for testing the sterility of infusion fluids. *J. Hygeine – Cambridge*, **74,** 17
13. Sanford, R. L. (1980). Cumulative sum control charts for admixture quality control. *Am. J. Hosp. Pharm.*, **37,** 655

14. Ausman, R. K., Holmes, C. J., Walter, C. W. and Kundsin, R. B. (1980). The application of freeze–microwave thaw technique to central admixture services. *Drug Intell. Clin. Pharm.*, **14**, 284
15. Walter, C. W., Pauly, J. A., Ausman, R. K. *et al.* (1983). Microwave thawing of frozen parenteral solutions. *Med. Instrument.*, **17**, 307
16. Holmes, C. J., Ausman, R. K., Walter, C. W. and Kundsin, R. B. (1980). Activity of antibiotic admixtures subjected to different freeze thaw treatments. *Drug Intell. Clin. Pharm.*, **14**, 353
17. Holmes, C. J., Ausman, R. K., Kundsin, R. B. and Walter, C. W. (1982). The effect of freezing and microwave thawing on stability of selected antibiotic admixtures. *Am. J. Hosp. Pharm.*, **39**, 104
18. Ausman, R. K., Kerkhof, K., Holmes, C. J., *et al.* (1981). Frozen storage and microwave thawing of parenteral nutrition solutions in plastic containers. *Drug. Intell. Clin. Pharm.*, **15**, 440
19. National Coordinating Committee on Large Volume Parenterals (1975). Recommended methods for compounding intravenous admixtures in hospitals. *Am. J. Hosp. Pharm.*, **32**, 261
20. Training Manual for Central Intravenous Admixture Personnel (1972). Travenol Laboratories, Deerfield, Il. U.S.A.
21. White, S. J. (1976). Pharmacist and therapist; synergistic action. *Am. J. Intraven. Ther.*, Oct.-Nov.
22. Skolaut, M. S. (1968). Long-term benefits of centralized IV additive service. *Am. J. Hosp. Pharm.*, **25**, 536
23. Sanders, L. H. *et al.* (1978). Evaluation of compounding accuracy and aseptic techniques for intravenous admixtures. *Am. J. Hosp. Pharm.*, **35**, 531
24. Dinel, B. A., Ayotle, D. L., Behme, R. J. *et al.* (1977). Stability of antibiotic admixtures frozen in minibags. *Drug Intell. Clin. Pharm.*, **11**, 542

7
Filters

The purpose of this chapter is to describe devices used for the filtration of parenteral fluids as they are being administered to the patient.

Devices which remove solid particles but allow passage of the fluid in which the particles are suspended are called filters, regardless of the shape, fluid flow path, or materials from which the product is made. Two basic filter structures for parenteral fluids are in use today: (1) membrane and (2) depth.

A membrane filter has a pore size which is designed to prevent the passage of a particle by capturing it on the filter surface. Theoretically, no inlet to passages through the filter is equal to or larger than the pore size at which the filter is rated. Therefore, all particles are captured before they enter the filter and remain on the surface (Figure 7.1), in

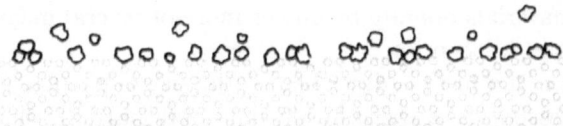

Figure 7.1 Diagramatic representation of a membrane filter

many instances occluding the passage sufficiently to prevent fluid flow. When enough retained particles accumulate and substantial obstruction occurs, the flow of fluid is impeded, and rate control becomes difficult, a phenomenon called 'loading'. For this reason the membrane filter is used most effectively when it is preceded by another filter to remove much of the debris in a fluid. In such a position the membrane filter becomes a 'final' filter.

A depth filter allows particles to penetrate past the surface. They become impinged in the tangle of channels that comprise a multitude of tortuous paths through the device (Figure 7.2). Only an occasional

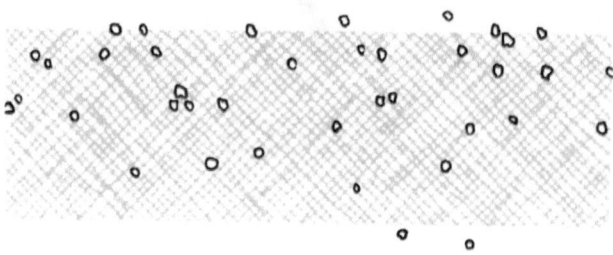

Figure 7.2 Diagramatic representation of a depth filter. Note deep penetration and escape of a few particles

particle escapes through the maze to reach the other side. The laws of chance dictate how often this event will occur. Because the filter surface does not build up a coating of rejected material which blocks passages, depth filters 'load' after longer, more severe use than their membrane counterparts. Fluid flow through a depth filter is easier to maintain than a membrane filter because there is more available surface. In addition to the mechanical restraint of a particle by a depth filter, another favorable property it possesses is 'adsorption' which takes place when a particle is retained as the result of attraction to the filter material rather than size incongruity. Many concepts have been proposed to explain how adsorption works, but no hypothesis has been proven. It is likely different depth filter materials operate by one or more of several means including entrapment and adsorption.

Performance of a filter is described by the size of particle it will retain, usually expressed as a percent of the total particle challenge. For instance, you may see the following statement: $0.45\,\mu$ filter – 99% efficiency, which means that 1 in 100 particles of less than 0.45 micrometers in size will pass through the filter. This rating is meaningful only for the test conditions it is reporting. Different upstream pressures, a challenge which is less or more particles, or a different carrier solution most likely will change the test result. If you will be relying upon labeled filter performance for a special application, learn the conditions of the tests which produced the filter rating. Make sure they are similar to your contemplated situation. When investigating a possible system fault, be certain to understand how the filter was tested before accepting its performance as stated on the label. Conditions in use may have been different. Also be aware that for a variety of reasons filters often perform better than stated on their label.

The primary use of filters in parenteral fluid systems is particle removal. Debris may be present in the solution because of one or more of the following causes: (1) solution–container interaction, (2) deterioration of the container or closure as the solution ages, and (3) poor manufacturing technique or raw materials. Pharmacopoeial standards have been published in many countries which limit the size and quantity of particulate matter in large volume parenterals. In comparison standards for small volume solutions, vials, ampules, etc., are loose or nonexistent. When the content of these preparations is added to large volume parenteral solutions, particles will be transferred with them. It is possible more particles will be created unexpectedly as the result of interaction between components of each container.

Lyophilized antibiotics are recognized as having substantial numbers of particles in many instances. When the drugs are reconstituted, the resulting solutions are particulated heavily. Some manufacturers of antibiotics that are especially noteworthy for particle problems recommend the use of a filter during infusion. Sometimes administration sets have particles retained in them from the time of manufacture. These small pieces of plastic may be washed into the patient if they are not captured by the filter.

The absolute 0.22μ pore size membrane filter qualifies as a sterilization device. This statement is true only in the specified circumstances stipulated by the filter manufacturer. In normal gravity driven intravenous infusions, conditions usually confer minimal stress and are unlikely to exceed manufacturer specifications. Presuming adequate quality control practices which guarantee the flow path integrity of the individual device, it may seem possible to consider employing a 0.22μ filter to administer a non-sterile solution. This practice is foolhardy in my opinion. It is unacceptable to rely on a filter to remove bacteria known to be present in any solution which will be infused into a patient directly. Some practitioners select a 0.22μ filter to sterilize an infusion against the possibility that a micro-organism has entered the solution unexpectedly. They believe this approach can reduce the incidence of bacteremia in parenteral nutrition patients, as an example, because these individuals are receiving a final product created from multiple admixtures which have a higher potential for exogenous contamination than unmixed solution. When an open, air-dependent container is part of the system, it is possible for micro-organisms to enter. To trap them before infusion, a 0.22μ filter is used by some. I have never seen data which support the efficacy of this practice. I doubt the concept of protection could be proven.

A final typical use of filters is to trap air when there is a concern about air embolism. Depending upon porosity (pore size) a membrane filter can prevent air infusion by producing an air lock through which neither air nor fluid can pass. Filters of more complex design claim to vent the air so that no air lock occurs. On occasion this claim is not entirely accurate.

Filters are stated by their proponents to have several values. Among recent and popular claims for these devices is they prevent phlebitis, the concept being that particles normally present in fluid cause non-bacterial vein irritation. There have been many studies which purport to support this view. There also are studies which refute it partially or completely. After evaluating several published papers, I have been unable to determine anything erudite or meaningful to resolve the dilemma. Certainly filters need not be used in a system that is to remain in place 36 hours or less. It is conceivable that antibiotic-containing solutions should be filtered if the intravascular catheter is to be at the same location for the maximum 72 hours duration. If you choose this approach, be certain not to make it a general rule until there is an absolute certainty no interaction occurs between the filter and any drugs to be infused.

A second alleged value for filters is they remove particles which can cause tissue reaction in the lung, perhaps leading to permanent damage. Research in support of this contention is nearly all from the animal laboratory; the investigations suffer from the usual problem of translation to humans where no evidence for the same phenomenon has been reported to my knowledge. If you intend to use filters to guard against this danger, don't bother. There is absolutely no relevant risk/benefit or cost/effectiveness.

Bacterial contamination is a concern for another group of filter advocates. They espouse the belief that filters eliminate the risk of infusing bacteria. Not so, unless a 0.22μ filter is selected, functions perfectly every time, and causes no difficulty which requires disconnections that can lead to touch contamination anyway. In my opinion, any vascular infusion that carries with it a legitimate concern for bacterial contamination should not be administered in any circumstance. No filter made in a mass production mode is sufficiently reliable to safeguard a patient. Wise persons would spend the money used to purchase filters intended to remove bacteria on eliminating the cause of fluid contamination. Prevention and quality control are more appropriate targets of benefit if money is to be expended.

Those who place filters in infusion systems to capture unanticipated products of drug interactions do not appreciate that particulate generated in this manner may (or probably?) signify one or both drugs have lost potency. Filtering out the particles attacks the wrong issue and camouflages the real patient danger.

When filters are used for trapping air, except in unusual circumstances, both the perpetrator and the patient are being lulled into a false sense

84

of security. The risk of malfunction in a crucial situation is too great to justify confidence in a filter alone for protection against air embolism. When a positive pressure infusion is being given, an electronic air detector should guard against air embolism. Filters are inappropriate as primary prevention.

Many physicians subscribe to the inclusion of filters for the administration of parenteral nutrition solutions, presumably in an attempt to lower the more than usual risk of infection. There has never been a proof these devices perform effectively for that purpose. As with fluid and electrolyte replacement solutions, more time and attention should be given to preventing contamination of these solutions than capturing bacteria before infusing carelessly prepared product.

There are several disadvantages inherent in the use of parenteral infusion filters which make their routine use inadvisable, and mandate review of specific applications before they become standard policy.

1. If the filter captures micro-organisms capable of growing in a parenteral fluid (Gram negative bacillus of Tribe *Klebsiella*, etc.), my colleagues and I have demonstrated a proliferation will occur in sufficient magnitude to result in penetration of the filter and release of bacteria into the patient when other than a 0.22μ device is employed. This phenomenon does not occur in 24 hours but can be noted in 48 hours. Even when penetration does not occur, there is release of endotoxin which enters the bloodstream. Quantities are small, but no one has established an upper limit of safety for endotoxin in blood; therefore, it is not known whether the amount released is harmful. It would seem almost better to allow for occasional entry of bacteria into the blood, relying for destruction on the inherent bactericidal property of blood, rather than accumulate them on a filter where they can multiply and become potentially more dangerous.

2. When filters malfunction, prime incorrectly or confound an otherwise simple infusion system, they are disconnected and reconnected or manipulated in a way that opens the fluid path and exposes sterile surfaces. These adjustments have the potential for inducing touch contamination. Without the filter the risk of this event is not present. Filters of smaller pore size have a greater propensity to malfunction.

3. Filters are inappropriate devices downstream of a pump. Many pump and filter manufacturers have designated some of their products (often those which are more expensive) for use with each other. They point out the pump will not develop sufficient pressure to 'blow out' the filter, or the filter has been designed in a way to

85

resist higher infusion pressures created by pumps. These statements often fail to consider the alteration in retentiveness which occurs in a filter when it is subjected to pressure. When pressure increases, pore sizes often expand, allowing particles to pass which would be captured in normal conditions.

4. Because filters tend to 'load', they have an increasing likelihood to obstruct flow as infusion time is extended. This event, which occurs as a continuum rather than a single moment in time, makes flow control in gravity infusions a more difficult task. Constant readjustments are necessary, and a satisfactory infusion is difficult to maintain.

5. Some drugs (such as insulin) bind to certain types of filter material and are rendered useless for patient benefit. Unless you have seen convincing evidence to the contrary, the suspicion for binding should be in your mind. No emulsions (such as lipids) can be administered through a filter.

6. At least some filters are expensive relative to their value and the infusion system.

If you plan to use parenteral fluid system filters, the following recommendations can form the basis of a policy and procedures statement.

1. The filter *must* be changed not less often than 24 hours to escape infusion of endotoxin.

2. Only a pore size of $0.22\,\mu$ should be selected (membrane or depth) to avoid problems of proliferating, then penetrating micro-organisms.

3. Do not use a filter in any system involving the administration of drugs unless there is written documentation that no binding or drug potency loss occurs. (This information should be reviewed by experts available to you in medicinal chemistry, pharmacology or pharmacy.)

4. Be aware flow rate changes will occur frequently when a filter is in place. Plan to give the infusion more than usual attention.

5. Do not employ a filter when a pump is being used for flow rate regulation. (Filters in gravity systems modulated by controllers are not affected by this statement.)

6. Be sensitive to the special risks for touch contamination that accompany the use of filters.

7. Do not use a filter to prevent air embolism.

SUMMARY

The purpose of filters which are designed for use with parenteral fluids is to remove particles that are believed to contribute to the incidence of non-bacterial phlebitis. They are not suitable for prevention of infection or trapping of air. Many of the values claimed for filters are based on flimsy evidence derived from experiments which have questionable relevance to the clinical environment. There are several risks and disadvantages associated with in line filters. A strong, explicitly stated policy should govern filter use to avoid significant problems and unwarranted expense.

Bibliography

1. Holmes, C. J., Kundsin, R. B., Ausman, R. K., and Walter, C. W. (1980). Potential hazards associated with microbial contamination of in-line filters during intravenous therapy. *J. Clin. Microbiol.*, **12,** 725
2. Collin, J., Tweedle, D. E. F., Venables, C. W., Constable, F. L. and Johnston, I. D. A. (1973). Effect of millipore filter on complications of intravenous infusions: A prospective clinical trial. *Br. Med. J.* , **2,** 456
3. Rusho, W. J. and Bair, J. N. (1979). Effect of filtration on complications of postoperative intravenous therapy. *Am. J. Hosp. Pharm.*, **36,** 1355
4. Chamberland, M. E., Lyons, R. W. and Brock, S. M. (1977). Effect of in-line filtration of intravenous infusions on the incidence of phlebitis. *Am. J. Hosp. Pharm.*, **34,** 1068
5. Allcutt, D. A., Lort, D. and McCollum, C. N. (1983). Final in-line filtration for intravenous infusions: A prospective hospital study. *Br. J. Surg.*, **70,** 111
6. Lukaszewicz, R. C., Johnston, P. R. and Meltzer, T. H. (1981). Prefilters/final filters: A matter of particle size/pore size distributions. *J. Parent. Sci. Technol.*, **35,** 40

8
Pumps and Controllers

This chapter is divided into two parts, pumps and controllers, because each device serves a distinct purpose and generally operates on different principles to manage fluid flow rates.

PUMPS

Pumps are in a rapidly changing state of technology. There are four basic design concepts into which available pumps can be fitted. Each will be described individually later in this chapter. Pumps in an intravenous fluid system serve one or more of several purposes listed below.

(1) Give more accurate flow rate control than is available with administration set clamps.
(2) Avoid or give warning about 'hazards' in standard infusion systems.
(3) Provide positive pressure for infusions into high pressure (arterial) systems.
(4) Initiate and maintain very high or extremely low rates of flow.
(5) Offer a mechanism for coupling to advanced electronic control systems geared to patient conditions such as closed loop feedback designs.
(6) Give potent drugs at specific and reliable infusion rates.

All pumps have several general characteristics by which they can be evaluated for suitability in performing particular functions. Two of these elements, accuracy and precision, often are confused and/or not differentiated. Each term has a definite meaning and describes a pump in a different way. *Accuracy* is determined by measuring pump output volume during a stipulated unit time, usually in several trials, and comparing the result (typically the average of the several trials) to a predetermined 'correct' value. When the experimental value is very close to the expected number, the pump is described as being accurate. Often the quality of accuracy is expressed as a percentage, derived from the equation

$$\text{Accuracy} = \frac{\text{Observed Value}}{\text{Predetermined Value}} \times 100$$

An obvious defect in this approach is that at high flow rates substantial deviation from pump settings will be reported as the same accuracy as small deviations at low rates. A sliding scale for reasonable performance, that is higher permissible inaccuracy at lower flows, is a reasonable approach to this mathematical aberration.

Precision is a statement of the range of flow at a predetermined setting exhibited in several trials. The number of such trials dictates the reliability of the value ultimately reported. For example, if in ten separate tests a pump delivered the same quantity of fluid, it would be deemed very precise. A reasonable way to express precision for pumps is to use 'Coefficient of Variation', calculated as follows:

$$\text{Coefficient of variation (CV\%)} = \frac{\text{Standard deviation}}{\text{Mean}} \times 100$$

Study of this equation will indicate that Coefficient of Variation describes dispersion of results around a mean (average) value. No reference is made to a desired flow rate or setting.

A simple way to remember the meaning of and difference between accuracy and precision is to conceptualize a rifle target with the usual bull's-eye and serial concentric rings. If five shots are fired at the target and a few strike the bull's-eye but several of the shots are in the ring areas with the *average* being the center of the target, the rifleman displays accuracy but very poor precision. However, if five shots are fired and strike the target in a tightly fitted group away from the bull's-eye, the result is said to be precise but inaccurate (Figure 8.1).

Understanding the performance of a pump requires an appreciation for accuracy and precision. Both are tabulated by measuring the fluid output of the pump over time. Mistakes may be made while doing these tests, particularly at low flow rates. The typical study involves collection of pumped fluid in a laboratory cylinder or other marked vessel. Quite frequently these containers are calibrated inaccurately. The flow setting on the pump (the predetermined volume noted in the accuracy equation) will never be measured correctly with such tools. Since the calibrations on the container in this example are fixed, the perceived fault will be one of accuracy, not precision. The best solution to this problem is to use a weighed (gravimetric) measure of flow, obtaining the weight of the empty container followed by the combined weight of it and the fluid. Making a subtraction of these values usually will provide a good estimate of the quantity of fluid pumped, subject to the mechanical error of the balance or scale used and reasonable skill of the operator. By performing the experiment several times at the same flow setting and then at other rates in the range stipulated for the pump, enough data can be assembled to understand both accuracy and precision. The importance of knowing these factors relative to intended use will be discussed later in the chapter.

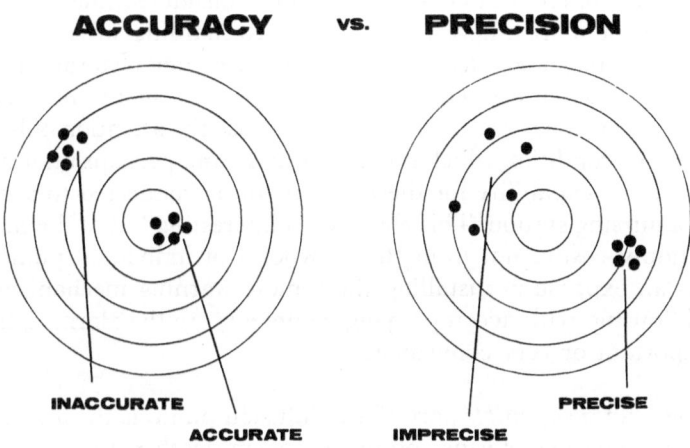

ACCURACY vs. PRECISION

INACCURATE

ACCURATE

IMPRECISE

PRECISE

Figure 8.1

Another aspect of a pump which has much meaning to the user is its power source. The typical line power available in the United States is 110 volts, 60 Hz. In Europe and the United Kingdom it may be 240 volts, 50 Hz or even something different. An adaptation must be made when transferring equipment outside or into the United States or U.K. Line power requires a direct connection to a wall outlet. This necessity is only convenient when the patient is in the hospital room, either in bed or an adjacent chair. Bathroom privileges represent a problem, and full ambulation cannot be accomplished while the patient is 'connected' to the pump. When the patient must be sent to radiology or some other distant diagnostic or therapeutic facility, the same power source problem ensues if the controlled infusion is to be continued.

Battery power is the obvious answer, and it has been incorporated into many pump models, particularly those introduced recently. Exactly how long a battery life is important is difficult to establish. A case can be made for 24 hours on the assumption that some total power outages (failures) in regions of the United States and Europe have lasted that long. These are very unusual conditions. It is questionable whether there is a justifiable cost–benefit for purchase of pumps with such capability. A more reasonable approach would be to consider the period of typical ambulation or the most extended time of absence from the bedroom by the patient for distantly located diagnosis or therapy. Using these criteria a battery life of 2–6 hours appears adequate. Often the range of battery life is a function of flow rate which can be adjusted for battery support episodes to the most efficient use level of battery power. For the presently available pump designs, excessive acquisition specifications may result in limiting the different models which can be considered, thereby risking the sacrifice of more important features. Recharging of used battery energy should begin *automatically and immediately* after restoration of line power so mistakes in estimating remaining battery life are not made.

The best pumps have several alarms to arouse the attention of hospital personnel to a condition which is extraordinary and perhaps undesirable. A few have the capability for these alarms to be connected to a central point at a nursing station. This elegance is interesting but at the moment seems unduly costly, not from the viewpoint of individual pumps but rather as an expense in installing the remote warning mechanisms.

The following, with accompanying comment, are the alarms I believe to be important or very convenient.

Air detector – an *indispensible* part of any infusion pump is the air detector mechanism. The major cause of air embolism death is the intravenous infusion under positive pressure of a relatively large quantity of air which subsequently becomes trapped in the right atrium and precludes blood flow through the heart, much like a vapor lock in an automobile carburetor prevents gasoline moving into the motor cylinders. At least one disposable cassette for a pump is claimed to be designed in a manner which precludes the delivery of any air beyond the pumping chamber. However, one death has been attributed to an embolism involving this cassette and its pump; others are said to have occurred. The need for an air detector is absolute on every device capable of positive pressure infusion, no matter how small the gradient between pump pressure and venous pressure or whatever the design of the cassette.

Low power indicator – necessary when the pump is in battery mode. This feature should be designed to give adequate warning about the impending deterioration of power below a level which will drive the pump adequately and safely. Approximately one-half hour would seem to be enough time for response to correct the potential problem without producing unnecessary harassment of the staff by alarming too early and too often. The alarm should activate when any of the critical functions of the pump may be impaired by a low power source (such as the air detector or speed control), not just the fluid driving mechanism itself.

Occlusion detector – to sense downstream obstruction to flow which cannot be overcome by pump-induced pressure. Several different circumstances suggest the need for this alarm, including a clamp left inadvertently in the closed position and tubing which becomes kinked as the patient changes position. This alarm usually works on the basis of increased intralumenal pressure in the cassette or administration set. The amount of pressure which will energize the alarm varies among the several manufacturers and is relatively unimportant (although sales persons will claim the contrary vehemently). What is more critical is the rapidity with which an occlusion is detected. This time depends upon the design of the pumping mechanism and the resiliency of the plastic disposable proximal to the occlusion. In several tests performed by my colleagues, it was demonstrated that a roller pump with no flexible reservoir responded with an occlusion alarm more rapidly than a cassette type set, even though the pressure setting for the alarm condition of the former was more than two times the latter. The reason for the difference was the roller pump had a delivery system substantially less resilient than the cassette with its large, rectangular reservoir. Do not be misled by simple statements of performance (i.e. occlusion alarm pressure is less for pump A than pump B). Test and understand the meanings of claims as they will be used in your applications. Engineering specifications often are not translated directly to clinical situations.

A confusion which occasionally arises is the differentiation between an occlusion alarm and an infiltration alarm. Infiltration detectors are intended to notice when the fluid being administered no longer is entering the vein or artery but goes instead into the surrounding tissue. Claims have been made for at least one device which will sense this condition. However, I have not seen the mechanism function reliably, even when operated by the inventor himself, and most users report they have abandoned the infiltration detection feature of the pump for which it was designed. Perhaps such a device will be available in the future; for the present it is difficult to imagine on what principle its function would be based, since several variables that might be sensed which signify infiltration are not significantly different in a normal infusion.

Keep open signal – shows a scheduled infusion has been completed, and the pump has shifted to a slower rate to maintain vein patency while waiting for a new setting. Keep open is a feature of nearly all pumps available now, and this indicator responds when the keep open rate is established so nurse personnel are aware of the change in flow. Be careful to select a pump that does not convert to a keep open rate higher than the flow setting prior to completion of the infusion such as a flow setting of 3 ml/hr that converts to 8 ml/hr keep open rate.

93

Prophylaxis is the best cure for problems of any kind, medical or mechanical. Therefore, hazard prevention should be an inherent part of any pump design, manufacture, quality control, and use in the clinical setting. The designer should probe for those features of the apparatus which, if faulty, could cause harm in some way. Either a fail safe mode or a redundant system should be designed for several features of an infusion pump. These are discussed below.

Excess infusion rate – In this condition the rate of infusion specified on the pump controls is exceeded, sometimes by a substantial amount, risking a significant fluid overload for the patient. A variant is the failure of the pump to switch to the keep open rate when a scheduled infusion is complete, leading to a potential for over infusion. Any pump suitable for clinical use should have circuits which can detect this rate variance and shut down immediately. An alarm should be signaled at the same time. The sensing circuit should be entirely independent of the rate control circuit. The failure mode should be to stop the infusion.

Gravity flow – Many disposables for pumps are designed to function with or without connection to the pump hardware. Often this feature eases the burden of priming the set and permits more flexible use of the equipment in keeping with the patient's needs. A danger is that the set will slip into a gravity flow mode unexpectedly if the pump hardware is not energized. Simply saying it can't happen does not make it so. There should be a positive mechanical (not electrical) control which protects against gravity flow at all times. It should be arranged so it is incapable of being bypassed.

Failure modes and effects analysis (FMEA) – The aerospace industry has brought to medicine this concept which is meaningful not only for infusion controls but all types of medical devices. The FMEA is a paper exercise, a hypothetical series of 'what if's', in which the failure consequences of each component are analyzed and portrayed. Those which lead to unacceptable results are re-designed or fitted with independent back-up features. Purchasers of critical devices in medicine should inquire about the related FMEA. The emergence of bioengineering staffs at many hospitals and their demand to review schematics of a device design is no substitute for an inquiry about an FMEA. A manufacturer which spends the time and money necessary to have a good failure modes analysis performed is almost always willing to share the results, at least on a confidential basis, with potential customers. (Note that an FMEA is quite different from a failure analysis which is an estimate of when and/ or how a device component will function improperly or unreliably.)

94

'Normal hospital use' – Nearly every device has a typical environment in which it is intended to operate. Much medical equipment is found primarily in a hospital, sometimes in a special area such as the operating room, coronary care unit, or emergency receiving. Infusion pumps seem to be used especially in patient care units where nurses seek to improve the accuracy, precision and reliability of intravascular infusions. Sometimes pumps may be subjected to an unintentional 'dunking', a deluge of solution or a slow, steady rain of drops from a container or set which is connected poorly. On occasion the pump, in its battery power mode, accompanies the patient on a brisk, bumpy ride to the X-ray department. There are several other 'typical' conditions during which it is reasonable and necessary to expect the pump will continue operation and emerge no worse for the experience. If the pump design results in a fragile, sensitive apparatus, even if satisfactory in all other respects, it is not likely to be a successful product or attractive to the user.

The best evaluation of 'fragility' or 'endurance' is a test in actual use. Before making a final selection among many different units available, have them tried in your institution and judge in part from the reports of personnel who come in contact with the device. Obviously, there are some events which cannot be construed as 'normal hospital use'. For instance, a fall from a bedside table to the floor below should not be expected to end with the pump unharmed. The classic six-foot drop test simply is not intended for infusion pumps. It is not reasonable to believe pumps should be designed and built to take such abuse.

Be objective in your evaluation of a pump. If you make unreasonable demands, you can anticipate the pangs of continuing dissatisfaction or, at the very least, a highly inflated cost to accommodate the special features upon which you insist.

Pump Types

There are three basic designs which are used to propel infusion fluid into the patient (each has several variants);

(1) Volumetric
(2) Peristaltic and
(3) Syringe

A final category would be the usual:

(4) Miscellaneous (other)

Some pumps are pure, that is they exemplify only one of the categories. Others embody some features of two categories as explained below.

The volumetric pump can be identified by the repetitive cyclic operation of the mechanics and a reservoir configuration somewhere in the disposable component. Commonly a mechanical arm is driven at one of many available rates, attached to the reservoir in a fashion which expresses fluid therefrom during each cycle. During another portion of the same cycle, the reservoir is refilled. Protection against back flow is provided by one-way valves that operate in a synchronous manner. The pressure curve of a volumetric pump is distinctive and may have a high peak to valley difference. Flow is somewhat pulsatile.

A peristaltic pump mimics the manner in which intestinal contents are propelled forward – by peristalsis. The basic configuration is that of several fingers placed adjacently, driven back and forth sequentially so that a wave motion is developed. When the last finger has completed its movement, the wave is picked up by the first, and another bolus is pushed forward. At least one finger is in a position to close the lumen of the tube (except in one design) at all times to prevent back flow. Refilling of the tube follows immediately behind the expulsion of fluid and is not an independent part of the cycle. Refilling usually occurs under the influence of gravity. Therefore, while there is a certain wave form to the pressure curve, the perturbations are more gentle and rolling, and the peak to valley difference is small. Flow is steady with a very slight pulsatile motion.

A syringe pump is usually a mechanical bed in which a typical hypodermic syringe is mounted after it has been filled. The syringe barrel is driven forward by a steady pressure from the driver device, frequently a latch or hook connected to a rotating gear. In this design flow is always in one direction. There is no refill phase so the pressure curve is flat, indicating a constant, non-pulsatile fluid delivery.

Readers having some acquaintance in this subject matter will recognize no mention has been made of another popular design, the roller pump. In the early days of cardiopulmonary bypass the dominant pump was the peristaltic model, but it was supplanted by the roller pump because the latter could be engineered to provide for higher flow rates and somewhat greater reliability (although I know of no demonstration of a significant failure rate among peristaltic pumps). The roller pump is a *mini volumetric* design with a peristaltic pump pressure curve. Distance between the rollers is fixed and similar for all segments; therefore, the volume in the tube between each roller is a volumetric reservoir that is propelled forward constantly. The roller pump has a continuous, one way cycle; it does not reciprocate (as in a car – combustion engine or locomotive – steam engine). There are no valves and there is no special segment of the disposable which can be called a reservoir. There is no refilling phase. Refilling follows behind a roller as it squeezes the preceding fluid embolus forward. The pressure curve is intermediate between the volumetric and syringe pump, having some suggestion of pulsation and a relatively small peak to valley difference.

The terms occlusive and non-occlusive at times are used to describe a pump. They refer to whether or not the tubing lumen is occluded or closed at some point at all times. Most pumps available today are of the occlusive variety, the closure being accomplished by the rotor itself or one-way valves. There are some which are non-occlusive, and these should not be used to deliver fluid against any counter pressure such as an arterial infusion or a known downstream resistance. The user should understand most occlusive pumps have the capability of building very high pressures. Linkages in the fluid delivery system **must be Luer locked** or secured in another manner to prevent unexpected disruptions.

Flow rate control has been developed in several different ways. Some pumps use a drop counter to monitor flow. For this purpose an electric device is mounted on the drip chamber of the administration set (*see* Chapter 2). A light beam is broken each time a drop emits from the drip tube, and these signals feed to an in-pump circuit with electronic logic that increases, maintains, or decreases cycle rate or rotor speed. Failure of the circuit to receive a signal during a prolonged, pre-determined period signals disruption of flow and sets a no-flow alarm on the pump.

Drop counters have presented problems in use including a poor fit on some drip chambers, additional set up complexity and mechanical and/or electronic circuit failure. Therefore, alternate designs have been offered, usually in the form of internal monitoring of the motor rotation speed. These have been criticized because they are an indirect reading of rate; there is no direct measurement of fluid leaving the container or progressing through the administration set.

Most people are aware rate detectors are available for blood flow in vessels; then why not for fluid in tubes? The reason seems to be cost. No inexpensive, relatively simple, reliable flow rate indicator has been found which does not invade the fluid path. An improvement of this kind would be a major advance to pump design.

This consideration recalls the issues of accuracy and precision, a concept that is understood well by only a few rate control afficionados and is abused by some vendors (in their advertising) and purchasers alike. Rate control performance should be analyzed and understood in terms of both accuracy and precision, and purchasers should obtain a reliable measure of each in an environment as proximate as possible to the anticipated operating settings of the apparatus. These tests are more important and meaningful than claims of the manufacturer or the salesman. Testing in the patient care area may show settings on the pump are incorrect (no accuracy, good precision) or changing plastic disposables might produce changes in flow rate (questionable accuracy, no precision)

97

or a varying voltage at the electric power source can cause changes in rate (unknown accuracy, poor precision, secondary effect).

To provide a simple means of measuring and recording rate control performance over time, eliminating the bias caused by several observers and providing a record for simultaneous future study of several products including the classic unassisted plastic tubing, clamp and needle, I have devised a test unit. It embodies a home computer with some laboratory weighing equipment attached. The system is portable so it can be taken to the patient care unit for testing control set ups made by nurses. A primary drawback is that it does not embody any consideration of patient effect on flow rate which is a factor in gravity driven fluid administration systems. These issues must be evaluated in a final test involving the patient.

Pump Selection

The selection of rate control apparatus for a hospital is not an easy task. There are several points which must be considered. Some of the most important are outlined and discussed below.

(1)   The purposes for which the pump will be used and its demonstrated and claimed performance characteristics should be correlated closely. If it is known high potency drugs will be administered frequently at rates which may vary among different sizes of patients or with changing physiologic responses (anti-dysrhythmics in a coronary care facility, pitocin), accuracy and precision should be key specifications. For administration of potent drugs where small changes in dose infused will have some effect on the patient, an accuracy no worse than ±5% of the stipulated setting should be selected. Rarely are such drugs diluted in large volumes of fluid. If quantities over 50 ml per hour are to be given, ±4% accuracy is a good target; when the infusion exceeds 100 ml per hour, ±3% is relevant and realistic. The precision should be not greater than 5% Coefficient of Variation (CV) at lower flow rates and 2–3% CV at higher settings.

When a pump is to be allocated to general floor use to manage routine fluid infusions such as parenteral nutrition solution, durability, simplicity of controls and portability (since many patients ambulate at least some time each day) should be dominant factors in the decision process. General floor use can accommodate an accuracy range of ±7–12%. The CV may be up to 10% for flow ranges of 50–75 ml per hour and up to 5% when 125 ml per hour of solution is being administered. Manufacturers who emphasize better precision and accuracy than noted above are exemplifying a quality for their product which is not an important attribute. Only if this improved characteristic comes at no sacrifice to other features (including cost) should it be considered in the purchase decision.

This relationship between purpose and performance not only impacts costs but also bears heavily on user efficiency and patient benefit. A pump without a suitable and easily implemented internal power source will make preparations to ambulate a patient difficult. If it is necessary to remove the disposable set from the pump to get the patient walking, the danger is clear. Another example would be the placement of a unit with marginal precision and accuracy in patient care environments where intravenous administration of potent drug was commonplace, a plow horse in a race for thorobreds. Equipment decisions can be made intelligently only after an analysis of intended use is available. Pumps are no exception. As discussed later in this chapter, a pump may not be the ideal device at all; a controller may be more suitable.

(2) The complexity of operation for any apparatus in a hospital is critical to its safe and effective applications. Training of personnel is essential. Too often pumps are placed in use with little in service education. Then, as new patient care personnel arrive, they are instructed by the 'senior' members of the staff, possibly someone who came last week and has set up the pump only once before ('see one, do one, teach one'). If a pump with many features (dials, alarms, indicators, etc.) is selected because it has certain desired advantages, plans must be made for a constant teaching activity. Personnel should be 'checked out' by someone who knows what the pump does and how to handle it. Complexity is a disadvantage when it impairs reliable performance of the user or the hardware. Sophisticated apparatus of any type may be a special benefit to the patient only when it is applied properly.

(3) Safety features tend to interact with complexity, that is the more safety, the more complexity. A good pump design minimizes this escalation in potential user distress by making safety elements an inherent part of the apparatus, not something the user must arm each time a usage is initiated. The air (bubble) detector is an example. When the administration set is installed in the pump and the detector is an integral part of the pumping head rather than a component which must be threaded separately, the design has served well to maximize safety.

(4) Maintenance of the pump in the patient care environment should be adaptable to any special requirements or conditions. If it is to be used in serving patients with transmissible infections, it must be designed for cleaning in a way which will prevent the pump from becoming a fomite, that is a carrier of organisms among several patients. The most accurate, precise, reliable, easy to use pump which cannot be cleaned fully,

properly, and efficiently has limited value in many parts of a hospital. This statement is *not* intended to mean the pump should be able to survive a 30 minute total immersion in a decontaminating solution containing 6 parts per million of free chlorine. However, its surface should be susceptible to exposure to a quaternary ammonium solution of proper concentration, and there should be no hidden crevices or corners which can become places for the growth of organisms untouched in the decontamination procedure.

Mechanical maintenance is the responsibility of trained personnel. A program of preventive maintenance and a method for routine checking of performance should be part of every manufacturer's package. When a concrete program which fits the hospital's operation (manpower, expertise, costs) is not presented, the offer for sale should be judged incomplete and rejected.

(5) Costs for pump hardware have risen rapidly in the relatively few years these devices have been available, partly reflecting inflation in the prices for all goods and services and certainly consistent with product improvements, sophistication in performance and versatility. When examined in the light of cost per day of use over a reasonable life of at least 3 years, presuming 270 days of function each year, a US$2000 pump has a price of US$2.47 per day. Extending the life cycle by 2 years makes the cost approximately US$1.50 per day. These are reasonable numbers and suggest even a very expensive pump is affordable. Initial price is *not* an important criterion for differentiating products. Don't buy what you don't need, of course, in terms of function or accessories, but do not downgrade a selection because it costs too much if it is the best fit for your purpose. A pump selected poorly never will have enough use to be realistically cost-effective.

The major factor in pump operating cost is the disposables. The price of a special set needed to fit the pump is US$4.00–US$10.00 each. Since sets should be changed not less frequently than every 48 hours (I believe it should be 24 hours), the disposable cost per day can be as high as US$5.00; these prices are subject to inflation (rising steadily with everything else), wastage, poor inventory control and other loss factors. Pump hardware which does not require special software is the most cost-effective rate control device available, presuming adequacy in other parameters. In addition, when any set from the general hospital inventory can be used, common established practices in patient care units remain unchanged, and training demands are not intensified.

CONTROLLERS

Many nurses would like to have a device that helps in managing nearly every infusion given to patients. The cost of pumps has been judged by some to be too high to accommodate this desire, and there are disadvantages, particularly those associated with infiltration of fluids perivascularly. Pumps can make a real mess in quick time.

With an eye toward these problems many pump producers began offering controllers, devices which were intended as an upgrade to reliable function of the sometimes unreliable tubing clamp and gravity flow. While the apparent problems in producing a controller appeared easily resolved by space age technology (if we can go to the moon, we should be able to control the flow of water into someone's vein), the real problems which appeared when the first prototypes were tested did not fall so easily to the innovation of the equipment designer. In spite of these difficulties several gravity driven devices are presently available.

An inherent characteristic of gravity is that it can be overcome by counter forces such as venous pressure which changes at the site of needle insertion every time patient position is altered. Therefore, as noted before, flow rates may change when the patient turns in bed, moves to a chair, or walks in the corridor. Little wonder, then, that regular infusions are frequently inaccurate. Further, it is not curious that claims made for greatly improved infusion rate accuracy and precision with new clamp designs are never realized in the clinical setting. The mechanical testing laboratory is not a good simulation for the patient's bedside. A controller, operating adequately, will provide one distinct advantage over the regular set and clamp – the elimination of over infusion or runaway.

A controller is an enhancement to the normal gravity driven *intravenous* infusion system. A special disposable is usually required for each set up. Its cost is in addition to or an incremental replacement for a standard administration set. This fact begins the cost-effectiveness decision process and has precluded uniform use of controllers for all infusions. To eliminate a device which can prevent an over infusion because of cost seems 'penny wise and pound foolish'.

The power source of controllers in most instances is *either* a wall outlet or a battery which is rechargeable. Hardware cost has dictated this circumstance. Therefore, a careful analysis of how the apparatus will be used should be a key component in any selection process.

A pure controller can provide no motive force to the movement of fluid. It measures flow and/or observes and moderates flow by changing the setting of an occlusion device through which the tubing is passed. Such a device carries no risk of inducing an air embolism greater than routine administration of fluid. Therefore, it needs no air detector. Because it has no inherent capacity to overcome any change in downstream resistance, the gravity controller system is susceptible to most of the same inaccuracies and flow failures as the routine infusion.

Beware of pumps charading in controllers' clothing. Some manufacturers have introduced a device they call a controller which can develop some positive pressure, intended to meet and overcome the variations produced by changing venous pressure related to patient position and condition. In a very real sense these are pumps, not controllers, and must be equipped with at least a completely reliable air detector. As mentioned before, infiltration detectors have not achieved a level of usefulness necessary for any patient application. Since these hybrids between pumps and controllers cannot detect whether increased resistance is due to true venous pressure or tissue pressure, such an apparatus can impose its own force, leading to a major infiltration if the latter is the case.

It is generally true of gravity controllers that they exhibit much less complexity than pumps and that, at least for the present, the hardware cost often is less than pumps. However, their characteristics and capacities tend to preclude applications which are for the administration of potent drugs, very low or very high flow rates, and any other but intravenous electrolyte and fluid replacement infusions.

SUMMARY

Instruments to control flow of intravenous and intra-arterial infusions are becoming popular and have increasing importance in infusion systems. There are two basic forms of devices, the pump and the controller. Pumps which provide a motive force to the fluid are intended to overcome substantial downstream resistance. They require several inherent features to achieve safety and effectiveness. Initial costs usually are of a higher order than controllers which are intermediate between tubing clamps and pumps. The controller tends to be less complex to operate but will not meet some clinical needs such as excellent precision and accuracy. Controllers will not *drive* fluid through an administration set.

The availability of flow rate control devices provides new opportunities for administering therapies which take advantage of special features in drugs, allowing the use of agents with a small therapeutic index and capitalizing on the kinetics of drug absorption, binding and distribution within the body.

In the future nearly all venous and arterial infusion systems will include a flow control device which is more sophisticated than the present day tubing clamps supplied with administration sets.

9

Catheters

The purpose of this chapter is to describe the structure and use of intravascular catheters.

During the last 10–15 years intravenous catheters have become increasingly popular. Their purpose is to establish access to the vascular system without using an indwelling metal needle. Proponents of catheters believe position in the vein (or artery) is maintained more readily than with a steel needle and less damage ensues to the vessel. While this theory seems rational, it does not recognize the traditional belief that metal imparts a protective effect to the immediate surrounding tissue which prevents the ingress of viable bacteria along the tract created by the needle from the skin surface to the bloodstream. Although there have been many studies designed to settle this and related questions, no consistent result has been documented clearly enough to resolve the dispute or characterize specific differences in the indications for use of the needle or catheter. There are few who would argue the issue if a catheter possessing nearly ideal characteristics is developed, the inference being that an almost complete conversion from needles to catheters would occur if some of the troublesome difficulties associated with the latter could be alleviated by design and/or material changes.

An ideal catheter would have at least these features:

(1) Easy placement and anchoring; convenient manipulation for attachment to the fluid administration set,
(2) Absence of tissue reaction for sustained dwell periods,
(3) Adequate rates of flow,
(4) Mechanical integrity; minimal frequency of leaks, weaknesses and other faults, and
(5) Flexibility for insertion at many different sites.

At the present time there are two basic designs that typify intravascular catheters. The most common is the 'over the needle' variety (Figure 9.1) in which a plastic tube is tightly adhered to the outside of a metal needle. The tip of the needle extends a small distance beyond the tip of the catheter to allow the sharp point of the needle to be used for penetration of the skin, subcutaneous tissue and vessel. The leading edge of the plastic is tapered; as it follows the needle, only minimal tissue friction is developed. Insertion is made in the manner of a needle. When the vein is located and pierced, usually signaled by backflow of blood, progress of the needle is interrupted, and the catheter portion alone is forwarded into the vein lumen and threaded in the desired direction. At the end of the procedure the metal needle is removed completely, leaving only the plastic catheter in the vessel.

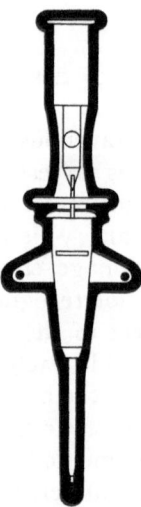

Figure 9.1 Over the needle catheter configuration. Note the needle protruding beyond the catheter

A less frequently encountered design is the 'through the needle' type. (Figure 9.2) In this device the catheter is positioned to pass through the lumen of the needle rather than over it. A disadvantage is the catheter must always be of a size smaller than the needle. However, an advantage achieved by using the metal or plastic protection is that biomaterials of limited stiffness can be employed for the catheter itself. These matters will be discussed in the section which follows.

Many different plastic and rubber formulations have been used for blood vessel catheterization. Changes occurred as new materials became available, were judged likely to be improvements, and were designed into catheter technology. Among the early materials were polyethylene and polyvinyl. They are easy to manufacture in several sizes and in

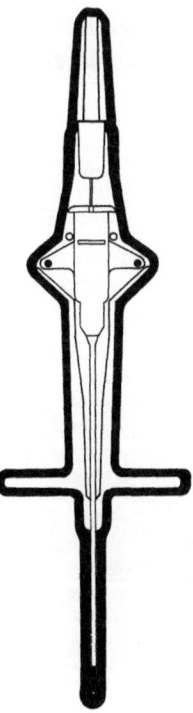

Figure 9.2 Through the needle catheter. The needle is slotted to permit its extraction from the patient after the catheter has been guided in place.

different configurations; thus, they tend to be adaptable to whatever use is desired. Unfortunately, each is inherently stiff and causes tissue reaction in the vein after only a relatively short dwell time. The patient experiences increasing discomfort. There is a risk of thrombosis with an accompanying (limited) possibility the clot can become dislodged and embolize. A more desirable material is Teflon. Several popular catheters are made of this material. It is more resilient than polyethylene and polyvinyl and seems to be less irritating. There appears to be a real increase in time between necessary catheter changes. Unfortunately, the typical duration of uncomplicated stay is still rather short, 1–3 days, a period which is not meaningful when long term therapy is anticipated.

Silicone rubber is a well known biomaterial which has been adapted to some peripheral vascular catheter devices. The fact that it is not stiff had complicated its previous use for percutaneous insertion. 'Through the needle' catheter designs have made possible the use of silicone which is judged to be non-reactive during extended implantation in tissue and non-stimulating to the natural clotting mechanisms of whole blood.

Characteristics of silicone make it an attractive choice except where intended clinical use is for very high flow rates or extremely viscous fluid to be infused when the limited lumen size would be a disadvantage.

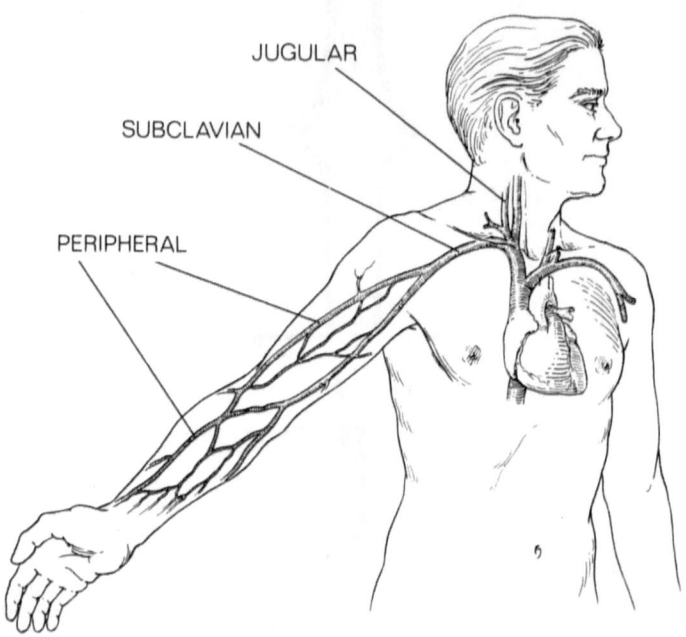

JUGULAR

SUBCLAVIAN

PERIPHERAL

Figure 9.3 Sites of catheter insertion

Any new materials should be tested for equality to or superiority over silicone. To use silicone, it may be necessary to learn somewhat different techniques of insertion and anchoring. Once mastered, the methodology is no more complex or difficult than any catheter insertion. An expected reduction in the number of catheter placements during the course of an illness and the probable absence or diminution in tissue reaction and its associated discomfort are advantages which will be procured for the patient by rendering such care. The burden of learning a 'few new tricks' is an honorable price for even the oldest and most tradition constrained 'dogs'. Unfortunately, at this time there are few silicone elastomer peripheral catheters available.

SITE OF INSERTION

Almost every vessel at or near the skin surface and several deep within the body cavity have been penetrated by a catheter at one time or another. Sometimes a great deal of ingenuity and a modicum of good fortune are necessary to activate a new infusion site in a patient who has suffered prolonged illness. In nearly all hospitals there is a special talent for handling such extremely difficult situations attributed to one or two 'experts' who are called when others have failed. Usually these people have a steady hand, a sharp eye and, most important, experience to fortify their efforts and constantly improve their skills. The lesson derived from this observation is that, as in so many things, practice makes perfect. A good infusionist will seize opportunities to make difficult catheter placements rather than shun them and hope some colleague will accept the challenge.

The typical site of catheter insertion for adults is somewhere in the upper extremity (Figure 9.3). The selection of a location should include consideration of at least the following variables:

(1) Patient comfort
(2) Risk of being dislodged during regular and abnormal patient movements and/or equipment manipulations
(3) Ease of insertion and anchoring
(4) Patency of vessel and
(5) Relationship of catheter size to vessel size

Years ago the antecubital fossa was chosen often because a needle could be inserted readily in one of several large veins which traverse that area near the skin surface. However, in every instance it was necessary to immobilize the arm in an extended position for periods of hours. Today this type of care is inappropriate.

Some infusionists prefer vessels on the dorsal surface of the hand where veins can be seen easily in many individuals. When sequential venipunctures are necessary as days pass, the selected location can be moved more proximally with a low risk of encountering an occluded vein lumen. Anchoring the catheter securely when it is placed in the hand sometimes can be a problem. Patients may find the profusion of tape and restriction of hand function are uncomfortable and irritating. Other health care personnel at times are confounded to some extent in rendering care when special attention must be given to avoid disturbing a hand bearing a catheter.

The upper extremity between the wrist and elbow is best as a location for a catheter. Veins usually are of adequate size to accommodate even a large catheter. There is little or no restriction to motion of the arm or hand. The catheter and attached set can be anchored securely. It is easy to identify the development of any tissue reaction to the catheter or fluid being infused. Local treatment can be accomplished readily. Many of these advantages also accrue to the upper portion of the arm. However, the anatomy of the area makes delineation of the course of a vessel in most people rather difficult as the muscle mass often is substantial and the location of the major veins more distant from the surface. Experienced practitioners will have studied the anatomy of the area and learned how muscle borders define linear fossae through which veins traverse the region in a consistent manner. Visualization or palpation of the vessel then becomes less important in making a choice for a catheter insertion site.

Special situations which attend the use of catheters in infants and small children are properly the subject of individual papers. It is sufficient to recognize different rules apply, and judgements are dictated by considerations apart from those of older children and adults.

A favorable trend against infection has ensued from the initiation of special catheter care protocols, typified by one shown in Appendix 1 of this book. Because the design of each manufacturer's catheter differs, it is good practice to read and understand the instructions for use which accompany the product.

It is not accidental that the forearm is much favored over the leg for venous infusions. In addition to the presence of more readily identifiable surface veins, the arm is associated with a considerably lower incidence of phlebitis. It is a general maxim that no venous infusion should be initiated below the inguinal ligament. Several studies over the years have demonstrated the wisdom of that rule for which nearly no exception would be judged reasonable.

INSERTION

After the site for insertion of a catheter has been selected, preparation of the area becomes singularly important. The purpose of preparation should be to make the skin surface clean, render it devoid of live microorganisms, and provide a location for adequate anchoring once the catheter is in place. Fortunately, these goals are mutually reinforcing. The accomplishment of any one leads to achieving the others as long as reasonable care is exercised.

The important word is protocol, a series of steps performed in a specific order that dictates the manner in which various parts of the skin preparation procedure and catheter insertion and maintenance will be conducted. Once developed, based upon some simple principles, the protocol should be published throughout a hospital and followed rigorously by all who insert catheters. Deviation or change without proper study of the possible consequences invites disaster in the form of an increase in patient infection, tissue irritation or phlebitis.

There are many good protocols for preparing the skin area surrounding the intended insertion site of a catheter. Critical to the success of every

108

one is the observance of an aseptic technique. Tissues should be treated gently. Hair should be removed by clippers, not a razor which produces skin nicks and abrasions. Scrubbing should be effective without being abrasive. A large surface around the site of puncture should be delineated. Donning sterile gloves is practiced by many to avoid the problems subsequent to touch contamination. (Some believe gloves serve the additional purpose of being a constant reminder the procedure should not be approached casually.)

As the catheter insertion is completed, there remains the task of anchoring the device so it is stabilized in a proper position, comfortable for the patient, easy to inspect while in place for proper function and generally convenient to maintain. Here again a reference to instructions enclosed with the catheter will provide a preferred methodology. Any significant movement of the catheter in the vein because of inadequate anchoring increases the opportunity for difficulties, including penetration of the vein wall and irritation of the intima. The application of tape on the extremity should not be circumferential, thus avoiding an occluded circulation. A good method for securing the catheter includes a means by which its full length on the skin surface from the insertion site upward can be inspected routinely. If it is necessary to unwrap dressings completely and potentially dislodge a catheter in order to look for early signs of a complication, the anchoring or taping technique is not adequate and should be changed. For the convenience and enhanced performance of all hospital personnel it is best to adopt a standard practice throughout the facility. The slight loss of freedom for the individual can pay dividends in allowing efficient, proper patient care. Catheter insertion sites should be inspected every 24 hours by palpation through the dressing. If there is a suspicion of irritation or infection, leakage or mechanical faults, the dressing is removed and unless there is absolutely no reason to do so, the catheter and fluid administration system should be changed. A moderate or strong suspicion of infection dictates culture of the *in vivo* portion of the catheter after its removal.

MAINTENANCE AND CARE

The keynote of catheter maintenance is asepsis. Recognize that the catheter is a direct route to the circulatory system and bypasses many protections against a hostile environment. The dressing should be adequate in size, dry, dirt free and secure. If it is impaired it should be changed. Several people believe the application of a polyantibiotic ointment at the skin puncture can be efficacious in preventing sepsis. Actually there are literature references which support both sides of the question of whether to use topical antibiotics. It is hardly likely an ointment will mitigate the consequences of an otherwise careless routine.

Accompanied by diligence and respect for the catheter and the host patient, it seems reasonable to believe antibiotic ointment, unless contra-indicated because of special patient considerations such as sensitivity, might enhance the entire protocol. However, some believe prophylactic antibiotics are harmful because they encourage the emergence of resistant microorganisms. Perhaps at some future date results will appear which settle the issue and give clear guidance. A few authors have suggested the catheter might be flushed at fixed intervals with a parenteral anti-biotic. One which has been recommended to act against infection by *Candida albicans* (usually associated with parenteral nutrition) is amphot-ericin. Unfortunately, this drug has significant toxicity related to its use. I cannot imagine such remarkable measures are necessary if all the other known components of good care are employed.

For several reasons it may be desired to use a catheter intermittently rather than continuously. To prevent clotting and maintain lumen pat-ency between uses, a solution of heparin (10–100 U/ml) is injected from a syringe equipped with a small bore needle (not larger than 25 gauge) which pierces the rubber diaphragm of a catheter cap. The solution may be renewed from one to three times daily, taking care to decontaminate the cap before it is penetrated each time. When an infusion is contem-plated, the cap is removed and a standard needle adapter is attached to the catheter in the usual fashion. A needle inserted through the catheter cap is not a proper means to infuse a solution continuously.

Non-steel catheters should be changed not less often than every 72 hours; obviously, this statement means moving to a different infusion site. Only in the very rare instance that no other locations for insertion can be found should this dictate be abrogated. In such circumstances there should be a good reason for not placing a subclavian or jugular catheter (such as a burn or infection in the area) before allowing the peripheral catheter to remain in place for an extended period.

Often a catheter is placed and used for a few days and then defunctiona-lized (capped and filled with an anticoagulant) but allowed to remain for several days. Somehow people think the risk of infection falls to zero if it is not used for fluid infusion. The contrary is true. I have seen several instances in coronary care facilities where an emergency venous access catheter is in place for 8–10 days. Because it is not used, it is forgotten. This and similar errors are terrible tragedies because they may result in a serious infection which is avoidable in patients who cannot sustain another insult to their physiology. To avoid this problem the date and time of catheter insertion should be noted on the dressing tape securing the device in the patient; similar data should be placed in the medical record. This date should be handled with the same system used for renewal of narcotic orders. An automatic notice should result at 72 hours with an absolute mandate for catheter change on the shift when the expiration occurs. This approach adapts an existing control method which is nearly flawless in most hospitals.

In the normal course of patient care the catheter will be removed when its convenience is no longer a useful part of the therapy program. As it is withdrawn, firm pressure is applied and maintained until it is certain no back bleeding is occurring and no hematoma formation (bleeding from the vein into the adjacent tissue space) is taking place. A dry sterile dressing is applied immediately thereafter, and remains in place for a short period of time. Culture is not necessary or cost effective in routine terminations.

COMPLICATIONS

There are several complications related to intravenous catheter use which have been described in the world literature. Among these are (1) phlebitis, (2) occlusion, (3) embolus, and (4) extrusion.

Phlebitis is the most frequently recognized problem which users ascribe to catheters. It is manifest in one or more of several ways: (1) pain, (2) redness and local heat, (3) inflammation, and (4) edema. Whatever the sign, the meaning is the same. The host tissue is exhibiting a protective response to an irritant, i.e. the catheter. Frequently the catheter must be removed in order for symptoms and signs to subside.

The causes of phlebitis can be divided for ease of discussion into three categories – physical, chemical and infectious. Physical sources typically involve the presence of foreign material in the vein which traumatizes the intima and initiates an inflammatory response. On occasion trauma also occurs when the catheter is inserted, and deterioration of the normal vessel lining structures proceeds from that point. In another kind of trauma some authorities believe insertion of a large diameter catheter into a relatively small vessel prevents adequate flow of blood to nourish the tissues and predisposes to inflammation and cell destruction.

Chemical phlebitis has been studied more extensively because it is easier to design controlled experiments which test the importance of several possible variables. Both solution pH and osmolarity have been indicted as primary causes for phlebitis. In several experiments where both were tested, only one usually emerged as the culprit. The difficulty is these individual studies point in different directions, leaving the student of this problem little guidance. At this time it seems clear osmolarity greater than 800 mosm/liter (sometimes less) will cause irritation manifest as pain and redness on the skin surface overlying the vein. The pain free duration of an infusion varies directly with the osmolarity; higher values will be associated with correspondingly shorter tolerance.

111

Whether pH is important has not been settled. It is not possible to specify a pH value below which difficulty is frequent.

What is clear is that certain electrolytes which are typical additives to infusions predilect to pain and irritation. The most prominent of these is potassium. It is believed generally, based on experience which is variable among patients, that a concentration of potassium cation greater than 20–30 mEq/liter will cause an adverse patient response. Several antibiotics likewise have been shown to engender the same response followed by frank phlebitis. In the latter case daily rotation of the infusion site may be helpful but is often difficult and undesirable. Instead, one of the alternate catheters discussed later in the chapter should be considered.

Catheter occlusion is bothersome for attending medical care personnel and, if handled incorrectly, potentially dangerous for the patient. For most catheter materials the tendency to formation of a clot at the tip or within the lumen is much greater if there is no flow through the catheter. Unnoticed interruption of infusion fluid flow may be the genesis of the problem. When it is desired that a catheter remain in place but devoid of flow, a preparation of the type described previously where an anticoagulant is instilled and refreshed regularly (heparin lock) is a good technique to practice. If an occlusion develops, whatever the apparent cause or circumstance, an effort may be made to clear the catheter lumen by irrigation with a syringe attached to the catheter hub. Only very gentle pressure should be exerted, remembering the mechanical advantage which can be developed when applying thumb force to the plunger of a small syringe working through a narrow lumen such as a catheter. If the irrigation is not successful immediately, the undertaking should be abandoned, and the catheter removed (a protocol using urokinase or streptokinase to dissolve the clot has been recommended by some). The obvious danger in this procedure is that a clot may be dislodged and travel in the circulatory system to the lung where it can form the nucleus for a pulmonary embolism. Another risk is that the catheter will be torn apart by the pressure. Some excellent practitioners absolutely refuse to irrigate a catheter with greater force than can be achieved by the solution bottle and administration set in the normal elevated position. While this view may seem unduly conservative, it has much to recommend it because it precludes embolization of a clot or catheter material. Withdrawal of the clot from the catheter is the desired technique. Prudent judgment would suggest careful consideration of each situation, guided by an understanding of the dynamics of the problem, before deciding on a course of action. It is always safer to remove the catheter and insert another, although at the time it may seem inconvenient for the patient and the medical team.

OTHER TYPES OF CATHETERS

This chapter has been devoted until this point to the most frequently employed catheter for solution infusion, one of less than 5 inches (approx. 12.5 cm) in length usually placed in an extremity. In recent years the popularity of parenteral nutrition has enhanced the need for access to large veins so very concentrated solutions can be delivered into high blood flow where immediate dilution occurs. The subclavian vein catheter is used for this purpose. It is usually 8–12 inches (20–30 cm) in length. The site of skin insertion is immediately under the clavicle at the junction between the proximal and middle third of the bone on the anterior surface of the chest (Figure 9.3). This location corresponds anatomically to the course of the subclavian vein. As the catheter is advanced, it traverses the brachiocephalic vein and enters the superior vena cava.

The subclavian insertion site is believed to be associated with a higher risk of infection than the forearm. Support for this concept comes from published experiences of septicemia when infusion is accomplished through a subclavian catheter compared with peripherally placed catheters. It is not clear if this problem is simply a function of different location. Instead, it may be the debilitated, often immunologically impaired condition of the typical parenteral nutrition patient is the factor that has increased the incidence of this complication. Much lower infection rates for subclavian catheters are associated with continuous anti-tumor chemotherapy infusion. Therefore, the problem is unlikely to be where the catheter is inserted through the skin.

For subclavian catheters there are several hospital protocols which mandate placement be made in an operating room, even for those which are to be inserted percutaneously. The patient is removed thereto, and all practices are followed as if for a surgical procedure. While this approach is not cited as an absolute dictum, it does indicate the respect which has developed for catheter complications and the advantages deemed to emerge from infection prevention practices.

The actual technique of subclavian catheter insertion will vary with the product selected. Instructions for proper use are part of the packaging in nearly every instance. The first encounter with a new product design should include reference to the directions which must be understood and followed carefully if success is to ensue. (The seemingly humorous phrase 'When all else fails, read the directions' too often is true. Sadly, sometimes we do not perceive a fault immediately and discover too late that complications have developed which could have been avoided by spending a little time in self-education.) A difficulty which must be kept in mind, particularly when called to see a patient in acute distress who has had a subclavian catheter indwelling for some time, is the extrusion

113

of the catheter tip through the vein or even heart wall into the thoracic cavity where fluid is deposited just as if it is in the vascular system. The first step in evaluating this problem is to obtain a chest X-ray, exposed in a way to enhance the contrast material impregnated in the wall of the catheter (a catheter that is not radiopaque should not be used in any circumstance), or injected through the catheter, confirming the actual present location of the catheter tip. This problem does not occur with silicone elastomer catheters because they are pliable and remain so over long dwell times. Originally supple plasticized polyvinyl chloride becomes stiff over time while in a vessel because plasticizer is leached by the lipid components of blood.

Another device, a variation of the subclavian catheter, which is intended to deliver the infused solution into a central vein from a peripheral insertion site, is the 20 inch (51 cm) catheter. The antecubital fossa of the arm is the point at which this catheter is usually placed. By one of several techniques, each special for the model selected, the catheter is inserted in the cephalic or basilic vein, through the axillary, subclavian and brachiocephalic vessels into the vena cava. Successful insertion of this device occurs in about 50% of attempts. It should not be left in the axillary vein if further advance is impossible. For both the subclavian and long catheters it is important that silicone rubber or its unequivocal equal be chosen to avoid thrombosis of a major vessel if the catheter is to be in place longer than 72 hours.

SUMMARY

Catheters as a means of obtaining and perpetuating access to the vascular system have increased in popularity and give every evidence of continuing to capture opportunities for use from steel needles. Although there are complications which are associated with catheters not found with needles, further developments undoubtedly will be designed to overcome these problems. Several means of access to the vascular system are accomplished with catheters that could not be managed by needles. These applications are important and useful medical techniques. Protocols for catheter care are necessary for the safe use of these devices.

Bibliography

1. Moran, J. M., Atwood, R. P. and Rowe, M. I. (1965). A Clinical and Bacteriological Study of Infections Associated with Venous Cutdowns. *N. Engl. J. Med.*, **272**, 554
2. Buxton, A. E., Highsmith, A. K., Gainer, J. S. *et al.* (1979). Contamination of Intravenous Infusion Fluid: Effects of Changing Administration Sets. *Ann. Intern. Med.*, **90**, 764
3. Maki, D. G., Goldman, D. A. and Rhame, F. S. (1973). Infection Control in Intravenous Therapy. *Ann. Intern. Med.*, **79**, 867
4. Simmons, B. P. (1982). Guideline for Prevention of Intravenous Therapy – Related Infections. *Infect. Contr.*, **3**, 61

5. Stewart, R. D. and Sanislow, C. A. (1961). Silastic Intravenous Catheter. *N. Engl. J. Med.*, **265,** 1283
6. Curelaru, I., Linder, L. and Gustavsson, B. (1980). Displacement of Catheters Inserted Through Internal Jugular Veins with Neck Flexion and Extension. *Intens. Care Med.*, **6,** 179
7. Hickman, R. O., Buckner, C. D., Clift, R. A. *et al.* (1979). A Modified Right Atrial Catheter for Access to the Venous System in Marrow Transplant Recipients. *Surg. Gynecol. Obstet.*, **148,** 871
8. Krely, E. M. (1978). Placement of Central Feeding Catheters. *Br. Med. J.*, **2,** 1123

10

Microbiology of I.V. Fluids

There are two unthinkable but nevertheless very real human errors which can be made in practicing intravenous therapy. The first is a serious admixture mistake in which the consequence may be a drug poisoning – too much of a potent medicine put into the infusion unit and then into the patient, or too little drug (perhaps none by an oversight) which fails to cover other medicine being given simultaneously or consecutively. The second fault is micro-organism poisoning, adding to the infusion system a bacterial or mold population which proliferates in the solution and is delivered to the patient causing septicemia and an entirely new and different disease process than the medical problem for which the patient is being treated primarily. This chapter addresses micro-organism poisoning. If you are not stimulated by the prospect of reading about little bugs that cannot be seen and surely will not confound *your* excellent practice, be aware that some people have died due to infection directly traceable to an infusion system. Do not relax because you have heard about these incidents and you know there were difficulties in the manufacture of the solutions that caused them. Contamination of parenteral fluids occurs much more frequently in the hospital and very near to the patient in the chain of events which leads to the administration of a solution unit rather than at the manufacturing facility. If you are complacent about the potential tragedy which can arise from small errors in technique, you are the person who can perpetrate one or more such incidents unknowingly. The purpose of this chapter is to make you aware of what can and may happen if you or your colleagues, pharmacists, nurses and physicians, are careless.

In addition to addressing people involved directly in patient care, other purposes are served by this chapter. It will be of interest to persons on the hospital staff having responsibility for infection monitoring and control, the infection epidemiology nurse and the physician infectious disease specialist. By deriving data from several sources, experimental and clinical, some direction can be given to the search for and prevention of single instances of infection and limited hospital epidemics which may have their origin in parenteral solutions and/or administration equipment.

For purposes of clarity, the source of contamination of infusion fluids has been divided into two modes, intrinsic and extrinsic. The former is very uncommon in comparison to the latter. Intrinsic contamination is that which has its source within the product. Recently, it has been identified most with faulty manufacturing procedures. These episodes tend to produce large numbers of non-sterile products with the potential for causing a nationwide epidemic. However, a more frequent occurrence probably is a single unit fault, for example a bottle cracked during shipment which permits micro-organisms to be admitted and proliferate. All of these episodes represent intrinsic contamination. Extrinsic contamination is defined as that which occurs when the micro-organisms are introduced from sources extraneous to the fluid. This phenomenon will be discussed later in the chapter.

INTRINSIC CONTAMINATION

The most obvious mechanism by which intrinsic contamination of parenteral fluids can occur is a failure to sterilize one or several units because of inadequate application to the filled container of sufficient heat for a long enough period.

The usual manufacturing method involved in preparing intravenous solution units is called terminal heat sterilization. It is the most desirable presently available method for sterilizing fluids, because from the time of completion of sterilization to the time of use the fluid remains undisturbed with no access of the external environment to the content.

At least one major instance of sterilization failure has been investigated and reported. In this situation the sterilizer, a pressure steam vessel, was being operated without necessary attention to details. Maintenance of the apparatus was below established standards. The ultimate result was that some filled bottles, placed on the lower levels of a transport cart in the autoclave, did not receive sufficient exposure to steam, and the internal heat of the product did not rise enough to achieve kill of all organisms. Some bacteria which survived proliferated and, when infused into patients, caused septicemia.

Having acquaintance with all the present major United States and many of the Canadian and United Kingdom manufacturers, and being aware of their diligence, expertise and devotion, I believe such instances are very unlikely to occur in the facilities of these companies. However, for steam vessels operated in hospitals to sterilize in-house manufactured solution, the complexities may not be appreciated or understood by the constantly changing cadre of attendants and maintenance personnel, none of whom can devote their full energies and attention to this extremely important device. With increasing pressures on the rising cost of medical care and government constraint on the purchase of equipment, steam vessels in the hospital are not replaced or modernized. Thus, they have a greater propensity for failure. Among the several reasons noted throughout this book for the abandonment of locally made solutions, improper operation, maintenance and replacement of sterilizers is one of the most persuasive. There is no greater evidence for the consequences of a sterilizer failure than in the United Kingdom incident noted above.

There have been four additional multi-unit intrinsic non-sterility incidents reported since 1970. Each of these was the result of a post contamination fault wherein the integrity of the container–closure system did not sustain the after sterilization intrusion of unsterile water. As these problems are understood today following intensive investigation, multi-material closure systems and the need to manipulate internal and external pressure in rigid containers at least were contributory factors. (see Chapter 2). Dixon has noted how minor the apparent cause of the fault seems to be, even in retrospect, and what major consequences transpired therefrom: 'This emphasizes how little we know about the many factors that influence the sterility of a complicated medical product'.

Another kind of post sterilization intrinsic contamination may take place much later in the relatively long chain of events between the sterilizer and the patient. If the glass container is cracked or the closure somehow is damaged during shipment or handling, there is an opportunity for the ingress of organisms. A proliferating culture of potentially pathogenic bacteria and fungae can result, leading to a patient septicemia. Of course, clinical evidence for an intrinsic contamination will be much less than in the manufacturer failure where many more than one unit may be involved. Diligence in prevention must be exercised by the nurse and pharmacist who prepare solution for administration by following manufacturer's directions for examination of the container and its content before delivery to the patient. Plastic containers are less subject to these types of faults. They have a small potential for leaks, however, and the simple maneuver of squeezing the unit just before use almost invariably will reveal any leak which could be a source of difficulty.

Because intrinsic contamination occurs before the final moment of use, the micro-organisms involved must be able to enter (or not be killed in) the unit, and then survive by the usual biological mechanisms of reproduction. Typical fluid and electrolyte replacement solutions have characteristics which form a hostile environment for most bacteria. However, it has been found that Gram-negative bacilli of the Tribe *Klebsiella* spp. do possess the requisite internal biochemistry and metabolism not only to survive but also to multiply and become increasingly dangerous.

119

As with many drugs, the greater the dose of bacteria the higher the likelihood of toxicity. ('Dose determines whether a substance is a benefit or a poison' – Bombasties Theophrastus von Hohenheim – Paracelsus – 16th Century.)

As the epidemiology of septicemias is being monitored in hospitals, the responsible individuals should keep in mind the predilection of fluids to harbor these Gram-negative organisms. Where or when an unusual increment in isolation of these organisms occurs, a suspicion should be aroused. However, when an infection is suspected to be caused by intrinsic parenteral fluid contamination and the organism cultured from the patient is not of the Tribe *Klebsiella* spp., other sources of infection should be higher on the list of probable causes. Clinical signs and symptoms of fluid related septicemia are not distinguishable from other causes of blood borne infection with the single exception that subsequent control of a hospital outbreak invariably follows the proper management of the fluid supply. Also, all of the characteristics of the clinical picture associated with intrinsic contamination are the same for extrinsic contamination.

Dixon has listed the epidemiological characteristics of a bacteremia epidemic caused by intrinsic contamination:

(1)   Increased incidence of primary bacteremia
(2)   No alteration in disease incidence at other sites
(3)   Single or only a few species of micro-organisms responsible
(4)   Unusual pathogen often responsible
(5)   Unusual and similar sensitivity patterns
(6)   Significant association with infusion therapy
(7)   Similar episodes in other hospitals

In every suspected intrinsic contamination problem investigated since these criteria were formulated, when one or more of the above elements were absent, the cause proved to be extrinsic contamination unique to the hospital and part of the in-house manipulation methodology for parenteral fluids.

EXTRINSIC CONTAMINATION

Extrinsic contamination derives from a source outside the fluid itself. The first such opportunity for contamination occurs in the use of most fluid systems when they are opened. Since all rigid containers are packed with a vacuum (negative pressure relative to atmosphere) over the fluid, the initial event attendant upon any manipulation is the partial or full relief of the vacuum. One study conducted in part to determine the potential for contamination of solutions when unfiltered air was admitted to the container during the opening procedure found that 4 of 16 units were contaminated with two types of 'open' systems. A rigid container with vacuum relief through a filtered air inlet and the non-air dependent flexible plastic system showed no contamination in comparable experiments. The obvious conclusion is that unsterile air has the potential for contaminating a previously sterile environment. The frequency and intensity of such contamination probably is dependent upon the amount of microbes in the air per unit volume (such as cubic feet) and the quantity of air admitted when units are opened.

A second source of peril to the fluid before it reaches the patient is the additives which are made upon prescription of the physician. Typically, these consist of one or more electrolyte solutions or medications such as antibiotics. Some large hospitals have centralized the preparation of these admixtures in the pharmacy (*see* Chapter 6 – Admixture Services) to achieve greater efficiency, provide better drug control, and place the burden of medication preparation in the hands of those trained professionally to assume that role. In general this approach has been very successful. However, it must be recognized that concentrating the handling of a majority of fluids used in a hospital at one point for at least a short time in the life cycle of each unit assumes the risk of disseminating the consequences of an error broadly and quickly, possibly in the form of an epidemic. Since central admixture techniques rely to some extent on quasi assembly line approaches to the handling of many units each day, a human error in dosage or contamination can be carried quickly to multiple places and affect several patients before the fault is discovered. One such problem has arisen and been reported with exactly the result described above. Sources of micro-organisms in admixture generated non-sterility may be either an unsterile additive component delivered to one or more units or poor technique in making fluid transfers. The latter should be monitored by a quality control procedure which is a mandatory integral part of any central admixture program.

Because of cost and convenience, many admixtures in the United States, Canada and the United Kingdom are made in a medication room in the patient care area, usually by nurses. Several factors may effect adversely the accomplishment of a successful admixture in this environment. These elements include (but are not limited to) a very busy and sometimes distracted nurse, a poorly maintained area shared for many procedures because of space limitations, inadequate equipment (the new syringe order was not delivered so we will use the smaller ones and make the transfer twice), and complex physician orders given without knowledge of and/or regard for drug and fluid interactions. These issues are addressed in Chapter 4. Those relating to contamination are suitable for discussion here. They include primarily poorly maintained and shared areas and inadequate equipment.

There have been several attempts to quantify the consequence of non-pharmacy admixture, mostly by pharmacists who seek to capture the responsibility for handling solutions and additives from the domain of the nursing service. (I think the latter would gladly surrender the 'privilege' – who needs more headaches?). The best evaluation available is by Kundsin, Walter, and Scott (1973) who conducted a continuous monitoring of in-use fluids. While several investigators have made short term evaluations or even simulations, Kundsin perpetuated her surveillance of intravenous fluids for more than 4 years throughout all patient areas in a large teaching hospital. Her data represent a true continuing situation (0 additives – 0·40% contamination, one additive – 0·78%, two additives – 1·51%). Her initial report demonstrated the sensitivity of her micro-organism recovery system. Extremely low levels of contamination could be detected routinely. Data from this study have reference to the plastic container only. Unfortunately, it is necessary to impute from the literature any comparison for data in glass containers, an extremely difficult and probably improper action in view of the duration, care in execution and established sensitivity of the Kundsin data which has a type of information and depth of study not found in other reports.

Another component in the Kundsin study is the subdivision of results into groups representing different numbers of admixtures made in the unit just before it was tested. There was an increasing percentage of contaminated units associated with increasing numbers of additives to a unit of fluid. This finding is not a great surprise, since for the closed system manipulation represents the primary source of contamination. Overall the quantity of contaminated units is very small, suggesting that nurses who prepared the solutions achieved a high degree of familiarity with the system which seems to possess features that make the adaptation quite easy.

A comparison with these data is difficult to cast, but one which has some interesting relevance was a study performed in another large teaching hospital in a different area of the country using the glass system from the same manufacturer as the Kundsin work. In a 3 day period 94 infusions were tested and yielded microbial contaminants in 10 (11%). However, there were no associated patient septicemias with organisms similar to those isolated from the infusion fluid. Typical hand contaminants, *Staphylococcus epidermidis* and *Staphylococcus aureus*, were involved 8 out of 10 times. *Escherichia coli* and *Klebsiella pneumoniae* were found once in each of the remaining positive units. Excepting the latter, the level of contamination was very low which is reasonable in view of the known capability of Tribe *Klebsiella* species to proliferate in parenteral solutions. In the experiment the control was the culture of 50 unopened units, none of which produced growth.

From the same study there were several observations made of phlebitis in patients receiving fluid. There were significant differences (0% *vs.*

45%) between patients receiving fluids through scalp vein (steel) needles compared to plastic cannulae. Antibiotic solutions were associated with phlebitis in 42% of cases whereas only 22% of infusions without antibiotics demonstrated phlebitis at the site of insertion. These facts support a view that types of solution *and* catheter materials influence the promulgation of phlebitis (*see* Chapter 9).

The most important lesson from this study is so obvious that it almost does not deserve mention. Manual contact with infusion apparatus by medical personnel is probably the major mode by which micro-organisms enter in-use parenteral fluid units. Frequent and vigorous handwashing by physicians and nurses cannot be overemphasized.

Several people have questioned the importance of air admitted to the container when egress of fluid takes place. A report on this subject concluded there was no significant difference between any of the systems in common use. One type in which air bubbled through the fluid without first passing through a filter did demonstrate a difference. This equipment is nearly extinct and does not justify the phrase 'common use' any longer. However, those products which are air dependent and use filtered air are subject to abuse, as they can be converted easily to the open, bubble through equipment. When the filter is wetted or the small ballbearing malfunctions on integral airway sets (*see* Chapter 3), there is a temptation to remove and not replace the filter cap. While the solution will run better, the risk of contamination is higher. The proper move is to change the set. Obviously, if no air enters the container during the course of fluid administration, there is no risk of airborne contamination. Even though the previously mentioned study did not demonstrate differences among presently used systems, in my opinion it is reasonable to believe in the superiority of non-air dependent containers, at least for the issue of airborne contamination, since there is no air entry and thus no possible air contamination.

Administration sets can be contaminated and remain contaminated even through many fluid unit changes. The work of Centers for Disease Control (CDC) personnel and others has shown how continuous seeding of the bloodstream with micro-organisms will take place until a set is changed. Fluid from a fresh bottle does not wash away bacteria in a nonsterile administration apparatus. Because of several observations made during the investigation of the fluid related nosocomial (pertaining to a hospital) epidemic of 1970–1971, a recommendation was issued for the complete change of all administration equipment (giving sets) not less often than every 24 hours. For the time and based on the evidence then available, this proposition was sound; it provided the utmost in patient protection although it was judged by some to be inconvenient and unnecessarily expensive. Cost and convenience are hardly reasonable arguments when issues of serious patient illness are being discussed.

Recently, after careful review of several prospective studies, CDC has modified its recommendation to a full change at least every 48 hours. This increase in time is not intended to mean all sets should remain in place that long; only those which are apparently clean and unadulterated with accumulated particulate such as from a blood transfusion followed by 5% dextrose should be considered for such favored treatment.

Personnel, particularly nurses and house officers who have the primary role in handling equipment already set up at the patient bedside, must be cognizant of the potential for contamination of administration sets. If an inopportune or unintended break in technique occurs, discard the set and use a new one. If significant manipulation of an infusion system is necessary and several series of disconnections and connections take place, at the conclusion of the maneuvers, change all the equipment, using the best methods while doing so.

Monitoring fluids throughout a hospital from the standpoint of contamination is the responsibility of the infection control committee and its staff. A simple surveillance of fluid use should be in place and fully operative. It should include the identification to the species level of all blood isolates. Data should be analyzed for patterns of incidence, in particular cryptogenic (obscure source) staphylococcus, Tribe *Klebsiellae* organisms, and *Pseudomonas cepacia. Candida albicans* is a common contaminant of solutions for parenteral nutrition containing amino acids and dextrose (*see* Chapter 13).

When pharmacy admixture programs are part of the hospital routine, a quality control methodology should be developed and sustained as a cooperative venture between infection control, pharmacy and microbiology laboratory personnel. These disciplines should review the data after an adequate sampling plan has been established to guarantee objectivity in the review is maintained. This procedure is not a police action. Instead, it recognizes the inevitable fallability of human endeavor and can give early warning about incipient problems before they affect the quality of patient care.

By now it must be obvious that prophylaxis is the least expensive and most efficient means of handling both intrinsic and extrinsic contamination of intravenous fluids. Particularly since 1971 manufacturers, with the help and urging of government agencies such as the U.S. Food and Drug Administration and the Centers for Disease Control, have adopted many improvements in their practices which diminish further the previously low risk of producing a unit(s) that is not sterile. For those few hospitals in the United States and for some additional centers worldwide which continue to manufacture solution on premises, one can only hope persons in responsible positions fully realize the complexity of the process and the need for great diligence. It seems hardly possible that in-house procedures could equal those of high volume manufacturers, but that question is left to the conscience of the administrators making such decisions.

For extrinsic contamination prevention there emerges, from experience and deductive reasoning, a checklist to be observed constantly and reported upon regularly. If a central admixture program is in use, note the following:

(1) Maintenance present equipment and upgrade as indicated by advancing technology. Evaluate proposed equipment for its probable effect on contamination potential, not only for its efficiency and throughput.

(2) Provide an intensive training program in the risks of pharmacy admixture with respect to microbial contaminants, their types, sources and methods of control. Emphasize proper technique as the *sine qua non* of a successful admixture activity.

(3) Design, install and maintain a quality control system. Consult a biostatistician when selecting sampling plans; understand the limits of detection for the system which is made operational. Consider one limit beyond that which seems optimal, and make a conscious cost/benefit determination in electing to stand at the selected level. Involve pharmacy personnel who function in the admixture unit in the review and analysis of data.

(4) Refrigerate all admixed units immediately after preparation, including those on floor storage. Temperatures at 3–8°C have a significant inhibitory effect on the growth of any micro-organism that may be transferred inadvertently. When contaminated units are held at this temperature, at least the dose received by the patient will be small. This precaution has little effect on contamination arising from non-sterile admixture components.

(5) On a periodic basis evaluate the system of preparation, handling, transport to the nursing station and storage thereon, and ultimate use to guard against insidious breakdowns in previously adequate procedures.

When nurse admixtures are the method selected, the following issues should be given constant attention. It is advisable to obtain consultation with the hospital pharmacist even if the pharmacy will not be the focus of activity.

(1) Provide extensive, in depth training for nursing personnel who will be doing the work. Individual nurses should be certified to perform the procedure only after receiving instruction and

demonstrating proficiency. Persons without certification should not make admixtures until they have been trained and qualified.

(2) Establish an absolute routine for preparation and administration of intravenous fluids – the 'protocol' to which reference has been made frequently in several parts of this book. Since many nurses will be involved in this activity, their initial in service training should include acquaintance with *the hospital* protocol. Absolute uniformity will not permit carryover from another institution where an individual has been trained or worked previously.

(3) Do not overlook medical students and house officer physicians who frequently can be the worst offenders. There is no formal training in a medical school curriculum for handling a parenteral fluid unit. Fortunate young physicians fall into the clutches of a diligent nurse who gives time and attention for individual training. Often, however, learning is by casual observation, hardly a substitute for the requisite formal education on such an important subject.

(4) Arrange for routine surveillance of all personnel who deal with fluids. This personal review should be random and at a specified frequency (so many observations each unit of time such as a week or month). A report of the surveillance should be made to the medical staff at the infection control committee level and to the nursing service head.

The final step in the prevention of serious intravenous fluid borne infection is with the patient.

(1) Include infusion site observation each time vital signs are taken, not less often than every 24 hours. If problems are noted which may have a source in the infusion or the apparatus, give proper notice to the physician attending the patient. Seriously consider discontinuing the infusion at that site. Where appropriate, obtain microbiology samples from the fluid and apparatus in accordance with the established hospital protocol.

(2) Be sensitive to complaints from the patient about pain, swelling and redness. Be over cautious. In the business of a typical day, it is easy to ignore a comment from a patient who may be giving the first notice of an impending disaster.

The final issue is what to do if intrinsic or serious extrinsic contamination is suspected in your hospital. These issues sometimes are not simple to understand, and even experts with many experiences find considerable difficulty in resolving every problem they face. A reasonable agency to seek for assistance is the Centers for Disease Control, headquarters for a group of experts always willing to provide helpful and considerate consultation. Their guidance can be very salutary in charting a path to a reasonable end point.

Great care should be exercised in attempting to culture either unopened solutions (with the intention of searching for and/or confirming intrinsic contamination) or products that have been through some part of the preparation or patient exposure sequence. Sometimes a true cause for patient injury goes unchecked because misleading positive results from infusion fluid and equipment culturing have suggested an alternate cause, the treatment for which does nothing for the real etiology of the infectious disease process. The National Coordinating Committee for Large Volume Parenterals (USA) (NCCLVP) has issued a statement describing the methodology for conducting such cultures. This committee was composed of persons from many different backgrounds and interests in parenteral fluids. Their guidelines for culturing represent the lowest common denominator of agreement that could be developed in a subcommittee which was not given the opportunity to test its recommendations and support its pronouncements with laboratory results. Too often such national committees do more harm than good by intruding into areas where experts fear to tread, simply because the committee leadership perceives a mission to be fulfilled and the authority to do so in a specific time regardless of outcome. In this author's opinion competent help from a single source, such as CDC, exceeds any benefit which can be derived from the untested guidelines for sterility testing publicized by NCCLVP. At the very least a hospital should obtain confirmation of its positive findings from a reliable second laboratory. Naturally, where false negatives occur, the motivation to get confirmation is very small but the problem caused by an erroneous interpretation evolving from a false negative can be substantial.

SUMMARY

Intrinsic or extrinsic contamination of presumably sterile intravenous solutions can have many causes. Beginning with faulty manufacture and ending with poor patient administration technique, nearly every juncture in solution preparation has the potential for introducing harmful microorganisms which may be transmitted to the patient during fluid infusion. Clinical signs and symptoms of this iatrogenic disease on an individual patient basis almost always are indistinguishable from other blood borne infectious processes. However, certain detectable microbiologic characteristics can be helpful in differentiating cause.

The most practical preventive approach for the health care professional and administrator is to insist on establishing good infusion practices. Monitoring the untoward consequences of intravenous fluid therapy can be helpful in early identification of incipient epidemics. The participation of the medical staff, pharmacy, nursing personnel and the hospital administration is essential to a viable system.

When monitoring suggests evidence that might be interpreted as indicative of fluid borne septicemia, assistance should be sought from experts having experience in these matters. The complexities involved in resolving issues surrounding such incidents require unusual competences which are not available normally at the hospital level.

Bibliography

1. Report of the committee to inquire into the circumstances, including the production, which led to the use of contaminated infusion fluids in the Davenport Section of Plymouth General Hospital. (1972). (London: HMSO)
2. Dixon, R. E. (1976). Intrinsic contamination. The associated infective syndromes. In Phillips, I., Meers, P. D. and D'Arcy, P. F. (eds.) *Microbiological Hazards of Infusion Therapy.* p. 149 (Lancaster: MTP Press)
3. Hausen, J. S. and Hepler, C. D. (1973). Contamination of intravenous solutions by airborne microbes. *Am. J. Hosp. Pharm.*, **36,** 326
4. Maki, D. G., Anderson, R. L. and Shulman, J. A. (1974). In use contamination of intravenous infusion fluid. *Appl. Microbiol.*, **28,** 778
5. Michaels, L. and Ruebner, B. (1953). Growth of bacteria in intravenous infusion fluids. *Lancet*, **1,** 772
6. Maki, D. G. (1976). Sepsis arising from extrinsic contamination of the infusion and measures for control. In Phillips, I., Meers, P. D. and D'Arcy, P. F. (eds.) *Microbiological Hazards of Infusion Therapy.* p. 99 (Lancaster: MTP Press)
7. Kundsin, R. B., Walter, C. W. and Scott, J. A. (1973). In use testing of sterility of intravenous solutions in plastic containers. *Surgery*, **73,** 778
8. Machel, D. C., Maki, D. G., Anderson, R. L., Rhame, F. S. and Bennett, J. V. (1975). Nationwide epidemic of septicemia caused by contaminated intravenous products: mechanisms of intrinsic contamination. *J. Clin. Microbiol.*, **2,** 486
9. CDC (1973). Septicemias associated with contaminated intravenous fluids – Wisconsin, Ohio. *Mortal. Morbid. Weekly Rep.*, **22,** 99
10. Steere, A. C. and Mallison, G. F. (1975). Handwashing practices for the prevention of nosocomial infections. *Ann. Intern. Med.*, **83,** 683

11

Patient Consequences of Abuse

The purpose of this chapter is to describe and comment on various infusion system problems that have a direct and adverse effect on patients.

While nearly anything can happen (Somebody's Law – If it can happen, it will), this text will cover four categories of difficulties that are prominent and frequent. Facts will be presented so a unifying conclusion can be stated, one which teaches lessons that should be helpful generally to all involved in patient care. The four categories are

(1) Microbial contamination
(2) Phlebitis
(3) Improper application of accessory devices
(4) Inadequate flow control

MICROBIAL CONTAMINATION

Microbial contamination of fluids, intrinsic or extrinsic, is so important that a separate chapter (10) has been devoted to it. Suffice it to say here that bacteria will grow in intravenous fluids (a concept not widely believed before 1971). Fluids can be seeded with micro-organisms at the point of manufacture. A much more frequent source is the hospital environment, including its personnel which are the primary mediators of micro-organism transfer from one place to another within a hospital. Hand washing, when employed frequently and properly, can do much to interrupt this transmission; it should be practiced scrupulously.

PHLEBITIS

Phlebitis is an inflammation of the vein (arteritis would have the same meaning for the artery), often without infection. The disease process may not be limited to the vein alone; it may involve the adjacent tissue as well. Because blood vessels traverse several compartments of the body, if infected they can be the avenues of spread between spaces which otherwise might be protected by natural tissue planes of defense. In addition, this type of infection can spill micro-organisms into the blood to be carried to distant foci. Therefore, an infection in or adjacent to a vein has the potential for making much trouble locally, regionally and distantly.

There are two types of phlebitis of interest to the user of intravenous fluids:

(1) Chemical
(2) Microbial

Chemical phlebitis is an inflammation of the vein caused by a substance noxious to the tissue. It elucidates a response of cells (seen microscopically, of course) which may be difficult to differentiate from that caused by other etiologic factors. The patient complains of pain, and the observer called to the bedside may note reddening of the overlying skin, inflammation (swelling, edema) and possibly a hardened cord indicating thrombosis of blood within the vessel. There may be a streak of redness which follows the anatomic pathway of the vein proximally for several inches.

Several classes of drugs are known to produce chemical phlebitis. These include some antibiotics such as gentamicin and tobramycin, several anti-tumor agents including adriamycin, and solutions of high osmolality (such as 25% dextrose). Some investigators believe very low or very high solution pH is a cause also, but there have been findings on both sides of the issue when it has been investigated carefully, suggesting an unidentified variable may be present and uncontrolled because its importance is not appreciated. More recently some studies have purported to show particulate matter in commercial solutions can cause phlebitis. The proof is forthcoming from an experiment in humans which interposed a 0.22 micron filter near the point in the system where intravenous infusions penetrated the skin. While the study was double-blinded and prospective in design, similar evaluations at other institutions have not yielded the same result. Also, the low level of particulate in commercial solutions seems hardly enough to produce the claimed result. I remain unconvinced about the value of final filtration for fluid and electrolyte solutions. Given the added complexity of the apparatus, it does not seem to be a wise or useful trade off except in special circumstances such as some antibiotic solutions which are heavily particulated.

Microbial phlebitis is a self defining term. It is an inflammatory process centered about a vein which causes the symptom of pain, and may exhibit all the signs noted for chemical phlebitis with the impressive addition of a hectic fever, nausea and vomiting. Not all these signs must be present to consider the diagnosis. Causes, of course, are all those things which introduce bacteria at the site of an infusion. These include contaminated fluid, contaminated apparatus, and a stream of organisms from the skin surface down the infusion cannula track to the vein. In some instances the source is intrinsic to the patient when a focus of infection spews organisms into the circulation; they may colonize and proliferate selectively on foreign materials such as catheters. At its worst, from the viewpoint of local disease, the formation of subcutaneous abscesses related to phlebitis may be seen or appreciated by palpation.

The search for a cause of sepsis (presumed or possible) should always include the infusion system if the patient is receiving or has recently received intravascular therapy. Shortly after major recalls of intrinsically (manufacture caused) contaminated fluid began to occur in 1970, nearly every patient fever was construed to have an origin in the infusion system. Often overlooked were simple things such as pneumonia, atelectasis and abscess. As with all investigations for cause of an illness, observer intellectual balance is critical. Intrinsic fluid contamination is rare, and infusion systems in general do not form a sufficient preponderance of infection sources to deserve first billing on the hit parade of diagnoses. They should not be ignored, however.

Another interesting factor to remember is that not all contaminated fluids, intrinsic or extrinsic, cause and produce phlebitis. Absence of phlebitis does not eliminate infusion systems as a cause for a suspected systemic infection.

The treatment of chemical phlebitis is quite simple – discontinue the infusion; apply warm (not hot) moist packs as much to relieve the patient's pain as to enhance the healing process. Elevation of the arm on a pillow often provides further symptomatic relief. The infusion, if necessary, should be started elsewhere after giving due consideration to the cause and taking steps to avoid its recurrence. An approach taken by some is to infuse the irritating solution for only a short time each day (when the kinetics of the drug predict no loss of benefit to the patient), using a steel needle of smaller than usual caliber such as 25 gauge. The needle and entire apparatus are removed at the conclusion of the infusion and restarted at a different location on the subsequent day. The theory is that a brief exposure to an irritant followed by a long period of rest can be handled by the defense and repair system of the body.

The steel needle, long an implement in infusions (and perceived by some patients as a device for legalized torture) was supplanted for intravascular infusions years ago by plastic cannulae. Practitioners thought several of the disadvantages of the needle could be overcome, but as usual, the patient has paid a price for the innovation. Lost was the oligodynamic effect, a property which imparts a local antibacterial effect unique to stainless steel. Through this means the track created by insertion of the needle is protected to some extent from microbial ingress. There has been some return to stainless steel cannulae with the adaptation of the scalp vein needle from pediatric use to general care.

Management of microbial organism induced phlebitis differs from chemical phlebitis in some respects, especially including recognition of its cause. Since systemic spread of bacteria must be presumed, it is often necessary to institute antibiotic therapy. It is important to include measures that will prepare for such an eventuality in the early treatment phase. Before discontinuing the infusion, draw a blood sample for culture from a location away from the infusion and, if possible, through the infusion cannula. Then remove the cannula from the patient, disinfecting the surrounding skin surface just before doing so to avoid extraneous and misleading contamination from skin organisms not part of the systemic process. When the catheter is made of a material that can be cut easily, handle the inserted end as if sterile, cut the tip off with sterile scissors, and allow the end to fall into a growth medium for bacteria. The culture should be treated like a blood culture in the laboratory.

Hopefully, at least one of these cultures will produce an indication of the infecting organism. In the meantime the patient should benefit from compresses to the area of infection, and the extremity should be elevated for maximum comfort. Often abnormal temperature elevations will defervesce spontaneously after removal of the infusion cannula, suggesting it as the primary focus of infection. Sometimes, another implant is the initiating site with the cannula only a secondary location. In such an instance most likely the fever and other signs of infection will continue. At that point cultures taken as mentioned can be an invaluable asset to patient management.

In recent years a relatively common practice has emerged which is designed to prevent the invasion of bacteria from the outside down the cannula track to the vein. Many institutions mandate the daily or every other day application of an antibacterial ointment. Once again there is more practice than proof. (Often, we are quick to adopt new ideas without convincing evidence of benefit and slow to test and discard them thereafter.) At least one paper several years ago demonstrated the practice was without value. I have not seen any persuasive information for or against the practice. It seems a potentially expensive practice if its value is unproven. Perhaps someone will be stimulated in the future to investigate the value of ointments in this circumstance. Some physicians believe this antibiotic prophylaxis may produce resistant organisms and render future treatment more difficult.

Another much debated prophylaxis is the use of heparin in the infusion fluid. It has been claimed this practice will minimize phlebitis, and there are reports of investigations in support thereof. However, other views have emerged which show that only thrombosis is reduced; the incidence of phlebitis remains the same. The issue is not settled.

Skin sloughs are a local variant of chemical phlebitis, resulting from the inadvertent and inopportune infiltration of infusate into tissues surrounding a vein rather than into the vessel itself. Some medicines in use today produce a very potent local effect. These include adrenalin and noradrenalin and anti-tumor agents such as adriamycin. The result is a chronic granulating open wound in which it is difficult to induce healing. Often a skin graft is necessary to repair the damage. When such medication is being infused, special care and attention should be addressed to the patient. Pain is not always an early sign of infiltration, so it cannot be relied upon to give adequate warning. My preference when these solutions are to be given more than once or twice is to administer them through a subclavian silicone elastomer catheter, maintained with a heparin lock when not in use. This approach may sound extreme, but it does avoid the risk of infiltration and provides other valuable patient comforts. Just one or two patients in your care with a skin slough will be very convincing about the veracity of this idea. Recent reports relating subclavian catheters inserted for this purpose to high rates of morbidity (infection, thrombosis) suggest to me the personnel managing these devices need to establish a fixed protocol as for parenteral nutrition. The fault is in the management, not the device.

IMPROPER APPLICATION OF ACCESSORY DEVICES

Our forefathers in medicine, if they returned today, would be astounded by the technical advances and advantages with which we ply our art. Almost every phase of health care has benefited; parenteral infusions are no exception. Among the simplest of gadgets we use are the infusion accessory devices.

For instance, the three-way stopcock has more applications than designs. It has not changed substantially since its introduction in the experimental animal laboratory, followed by migration to the operating theater where the anesthesiologist found it to be an implement of uncommon virtuosity. It permitted switching and cycling of several fluids such as saline and blood. When connected in sequence (several in a row), taps to the primary line were nearly endless and provided an attractive opportunity for pharmacologic manipulation of the patient's physiology. The limit was the skill of the anesthesiologist to turn the levers in the proper manner so the liquid, whatever it was, flowed into the proper part of the system. Since most anesthesiologists are 'physiologic mechanics', the challenge was easy to manage, and the practice of using three way access devices burgeoned without thought for the problems which were introduced.

In our plastic disposable world the metal stopcock which was difficult to maintain and sterilize (therefore dangerous to the patient) has been replaced by a single use, disposable product. The problem is the definition of single use which is taken to mean by many that it is for a single patient – forever. While we busy ourselves changing fluid containers and even administration sets, the three way stopcock remains imperiously in place, resisting the advances of all but the most concerned until the infusion system of which it is part is discontinued permanently.

The stopcock provides the easiest access to the patient for infecting bacteria of any infusion equipment available. Its many separate limbs are readily accessible points for touch contamination. They are almost always wet, and bacteria have a fertile place to reside until they are swept into the fluid stream as the source of infusate is changed. Several studies have shown up to 50% contamination with common skin organisms among large samples of in use three way stopcocks. Since the stopcock seems to be an absolute necessity to perform our duties properly, a few simple concepts may prevent its conversion to a deadly nidus of infection:

(1) Avoid touch contamination of the limbs not in use – cover them with a sterile device made for the purpose.

(2) Do not use stopcocks as a multiplexed sequence of two or more. Mistakes in setting flow patterns lead to inward migration of bacteria.

(3) Use a stopcock only when absolutely necessary – they are potentially dangerous tools.

(4) Remove stopcocks immediately when they are no longer needed – change the entire system with which they are associated not less frequently than every 24 hours – have a routine for doing so that everyone can follow easily (such as all stopcocks will be changed at hour x each day).

Central venous pressure apparatus is another of the accessory devices which provide direct access to the vascular system. Its use has become so common that its complexity and danger are disdained. As it is manipulated frequently, it is an important source of contamination. People who touch the device 'just to make it a little more accurate' somehow do not feel the need to practice handwashing, etc. The central venous pressure manometer and the associated fluid path deserve respect. The assemblage must be used with care. Physicians should understand it is an ever present source of infection. It should be ordered taken down when its value is minimal or non-existent in a given patient. Nurses should remind physicians when it seems CVP measurements may have outlived their usefulness for a patient.

Of course there are many accessories which have not been discussed or even mentioned. An important concept to be appreciated is that the introduction of any 'special feature' to an infusion system enhances its complexity and thereby its risk for doing harm.

INADEQUATE FLOW CONTROL

Most nurses would say the single most troublesome element in any infusion system is flow control. Fluid comes forth from its container either as a waterfall or a trickle with few intermediate gradations. The system has a mind of its own, selecting that flow rate seemingly calculated to be exactly opposite to what is desired and intended specifically to embarrass the nurse charged with meeting physician orders. In general, I would agree with this assessment. Physicians know how hard it is to control flow rates, but few are willing to accept excuses when it appears orders are not followed to the letter. On the other side I have no patience for the nurse who operates with the 'set it and forget it' philosophy who returns to the bedside hours later to find a 'surprise'. Nurses know better, and they should expect to manage an infusion just as well as other functions in the total care of the patient.

While a simple gravity induced flow system should be easy to control, as changes in tubing have come forward from multiple use latex to single use polyvinyl chloride, the principles attendant upon control by a clamp have become increasingly complex. In actual fact it is mostly one feature of polyvinyl chloride tubing that makes it so difficult to manage: the tendency to take a 'set' or 'cold flow' which alters its configuration from time to time with seemingly no outside intervention. This statement should not be interpreted as indicating PVC tubing has a mind of its own. In actual fact it is the force of changes in flow we attempt to make which leads to further alterations in the internal lumen configuration and more flow rate changes than desired.

To be master of the situation instead of its slave, appreciate these facts and return to the patient often, especially in the first hour or two of an infusion. Do *not* set a rate which will compensate for what you think *will* happen; it won't much of the time. Be grateful that for the most part the tendency to further change in rate will be to the lower flows, thereby protecting the patient from runaways. Understand that when a patient moves from a reclining position to sitting in a chair there will be rate changes. When you assist the patient down the corridor for much needed ambulation, expect the rate to have changed by the time you return. In each of these circumstances you have changed conditions which influence the infusion rate.

There are several major factors which can modify flow rate other than the mechanical features of PVC tubing. These include the following:

(1) Change in venous pressure – caused by positional change of the patient (see text)
(2) Change in position, particularly the height, of the fluid container
(3) Clot forming in the cannula
(4) Filter loading, plugging or change in functional flow path of accessory devices
(5) Clamp malfunction

It has been popular to rest the heaviest blame for flow control difficulties on alterations in patient venous pressure. A recent sophisticated study teaches otherwise, and the dominance of thinking on this subject may be changing to other factors.

If you understand what might be causing a problem with a particular infusion, you will be equipped to develop a remedy. The list above is helpful as a reminder of what to look for when an infusion is giving more than usual difficulty.

For flow control the most dangerous difficulty is overinfusion, too much fluid too quickly. It can lead to irreversible pulmonary edema and death. Lesser consequences include right heart strain and interstitial tissue edema in some circumstances. Overinfusion recognized in its incipient state usually results in compensatory slowing of the infusion with all of the problems associated with resetting flow rates. Another consequence of overinfusion can be the delivery of excess medication if the infusion solution is being used for more than fluid or electrolyte replacement. There are several drugs delivered by the parenteral route which can be toxic if excessive blood levels are reached. When overinfusion occurs, these levels may rise rapidly with consequent potential for toxicity.

Underinfusion seems less of a potential patient hazard. Admittedly, it is more subtle in its consequences, but danger to the patient is very real. When it occurs chronically, dehydration can develop. The natural response to underinfusion is to increase the rate above its prescribed limits with the subsequent risk of overinfusion. Finally, when medication is involved, an adequate constant blood level may not be achieved, leading to the emergence of antibiotic resistant micro-organisms or the false conclusion of disease resistant treatment which can lead to an unnecessary change in therapy.

One often used means to combat these problems, especially overinfusion, is to interpose a secondary container (Buretrol, etc.) in the system, thought to be advantageous because the amount of fluid available for immediate infusion is limited to quantities less than the primary container. While this statement is true, these devices add needlessly to the complexity of an infusion. Also, they confound an already difficult situation by changing the functional head of pressure, making rate setting a real problem indeed. Some investigators have shown there are missed drug doses with secondary containers, and the persistent threat of contamination is obvious. These devices were designed originally to increase the accuracy of measurement of fluid volume, especially for pediatric units where ±10 ml can make a difference. They should be employed for such purposes only.

Mechanical pumps have taken a place in infusion rate control which can minimize the disasters of over and under infusion quite nicely. In my opinion they should be available at every bedside, not just in intensive care units or other critical care areas. I believe they have reached a level of sufficient sophistication and reliability to justify such broad use. As we give more medication intravenously and intra-arterially, pumps become important adjuncts. For convenience and economy I favor devices which use standard administration sets.

Present day controllers only protect against overinfusion (*see* chapter 8). They are not sufficiently valuable to support widespread use in a hospital in my opinion, even though the acquisition cost may be less.

While the dream of electromechanical rate control for every hospital bed may be materializing, those who remain burdened with lesser systems will do well to remember that over-compensation for underinfusion or overinfusion 'to catch up' can lead to grievous consequences for the patient. All the explanations you can muster will be unsatisfactory if an adverse patient reaction occurs. Be even handed and even tempered in managing parenteral infusions.

This chapter is not intended to be a comprehensive recitation of all problems which can arise during the use of intravascular fluid administration systems. Some common problems have been discussed to demonstrate two critical points when selecting and implementing a parenteral infusion and the associated hardware and disposables:

(1) Use the most simple assemblage of devices and disposables possible to accomplish the assigned task.
(2) Be familiar with the equipment and supplies you select.

Abramson *et al.* have reported experience in a busy university intensive care unit, an environment where problems are not unexpected because of the grave illness of the patients and the complicated care being given. Of 92 incident reports categorized as related to human error, there were 7 (8%) attributable to intravenous fluids. Aberrant episodes in the equipment category included 12 involving infusion pumps and 16 related to intravascular catheters, representing a total of 78%. These are not comforting data. They show much improvement can be made in intravascular infusions to enhance patient safety.

Of equal interest in this report was the fact that 25% of the incidents occurred during July and August, one-fourth of the problems in one-sixth of the year. The timing and quantity of these problems correlate with a greater population of inexperienced personnel on hospital staffs at that time of year. These facts teach a lesson which should be remembered and respected by all.

IF YOU DON'T UNDERSTAND WITH WHAT YOU ARE WORKING, DO NOT PROCEED UNTIL YOU HAVE HELP THAT DOES.

Ours is an apprenticeship art. It is not an embarrassment or sign of incompetence to request assistance in performing a duty. Similarly, help should be given freely and in full measure by those who are capable. As our calling evolves into ever more complex functions and super specialties, learning from others will make your work better and more personally rewarding.

SUMMARY

Fluid systems can be mishandled to the detriment of the patient. Reasonable care and proper understanding of apparatus will protect against the majority of mishaps. Even the most experienced among us can be a beginner for new technologies. Ask for assistance when you need it; give help and guidance when you are qualified. It is the tradition of our profession to do so.

Bibliography

1. Shapiro, S., Slone, D., Lewis, G. P. and Jeck, H. (1971). Fatal drug reactions among medical inpatients. *J. Am. Med. Assoc.*, **216,** 467
2. Gaze, N. R. (1978). Tissue necrosis caused by commonly used intravenous infusions. *Lancet*, **2,** 417
3. Abramson, N. S., Wald, K. S., Grevik, A. N. A., *et al.* (1980). Adverse occurrences in intensive care units. *J. Am. Med. Assoc.*, **244,** 1582
4. Chaput de Saintonge, D. M. and Newman, M. S. (1974). Variation in intravenous infusion rates. *Br. Med. J.*, **4,** 532.
5. Clarke, E. W., Jamison, J. P. and Quartey-Papafio, J. B. (1979). Impairment of flow in routine gravity-fed intravenous infusions in surgical patients. *Clin. Sci.*, **57,** 515
6. Dryden, G. E. and Brickler, J. (1979). Stopcock contamination. *Anesth. Analg.*, **58,** 141
7. Oberhammer, E. P. (1980). Contamination of injection ports on intravenous cannulae. *Lancet*, **2,** 1027

12

Blood Administration Systems

Note – It has been my privilege for several years to have an association with two men who were involved in the conception and evolution of the plastic blood container. This chapter is dedicated with respect and admiration to Messrs Carl W. Walter, MD, Emeritus Clinical Professor of Surgery, Harvard University, and David Bellamy, Jr., Vice President – Technical Administration, Baxter Travenol Laboratories, honoring their work to create a medical revolution from which all mankind has benefited. Those who remember the era of the glass blood collection container will appreciate the meaning of these words.

HISTORY OF BLOOD TRANSFUSION

Readers of Chapter 1 will recognize the name of Christopher Wren, astronomer, mathematician and architect, as the first person to administer an intravenous infusion (1656). A disciple of Wren, Richard Lower, performed the first transfusion of blood in experiments suggested by Wren (1665). Lower demonstrated the transfer of blood from the carotid artery of one dog into the jugular vein of another through a series of connected quills. Previously, in 1658, Denis, a physician at the court of Louis XIV, had transfused lamb's blood into a youth. Having met with apparent success in treating this first patient, Denis undertook several others with a much less satisfactory result. (This example is classic for medical science; the first patient subjected to a new therapy seemingly does well; additions to the series frequently fare poorly.)

For more than a century thereafter no useful improvement occurred in the state of knowledge about blood transfusion. Then in 1818 Blundell, in London, successfully transfused moribund women who suffered puerperal hemorrhage. When post-operative sepsis was controlled by

139

pre-operative and peri-operative antiseptic measures ('Now we wash our hands *before* surgery' – Bergmann, 1882), hemorrhage and shock became the primary mediators of death following surgery, and transfusion was attempted to treat this problem. Differences among bloods from several human sources (blood types) were demonstrated in 1900 (Landsteiner). Less than 10 years later blood transfusions were being performed frequently.

During World War I direct person to person transfer of blood was supplanted by the discovery that sodium citrate would prevent *ex vivo* clotting. Blood could then be stored, resulting in the birth of blood banks.

History has seen trials of many blood substitutes. However, only volume replacement can be accomplished routinely with artificial materials. Other special characteristics of blood (clotting, oxygen transfer, pH control and carbon dioxide elimination) have not been simulated adequately in a single solution. In a few cases patients have refused blood on religious grounds and were given a fluorinated compound capable of conveying oxygen in a crude manner. The development of very sophisticated techniques for obtaining, storing, organizing, dispensing and administering whole blood and its components may have made the search for a suitable blood substitute more academic than practical at least for non military purposes. At present the quest does not appear to be economically realistic. An important motivation for seeking a non-natural substitute is the avoidance of transfusion associated hepatitis. Vaccination and pretransfusion testing of donated units has supervened some of this risk already.

Blood is an amazingly complex material. Substantial differences between it and infusion fluids require unique techniques in handling and administration.

Glass was the original container chosen for storage of donated blood. It has been supplanted almost entirely by the plastic container which has benefits such as a closed system, opportunities for separation and individual use of blood components, and safe extended storage conditions. Too many years have passed since plastic units replaced glass containers to justify any description of the latter.

DESCRIPTION OF THE SYSTEM

An entire blood transfusion system includes three major elements: (1) removal from the donor, (2) storage and processing, and (3) administration to recipients. The technology associated with each element is extensive. Since this book deals primarily with infusions, only the administration portion of the blood system will be discussed.

A unit of whole blood is collected, stored and dispensed in the same container. When donated whole blood is separated into components, every effort is made to maintain a closed system with no intrusion of the outside environment which might render the product inherently dangerous rather than life saving.

Container

The plastic container, called a blood pack, is the heart of the system. It will not break, does not require admission of air during use, and has no closures or seals made of a different material than the main body of the container. The shape of a blood pack is not a coincidence. It has a 'dome' configuration (Figure 12.1) which directs fluid flow toward the outlet ports, facilitating complete drainage of the content during transfusion and removal of plasma during component preparation.

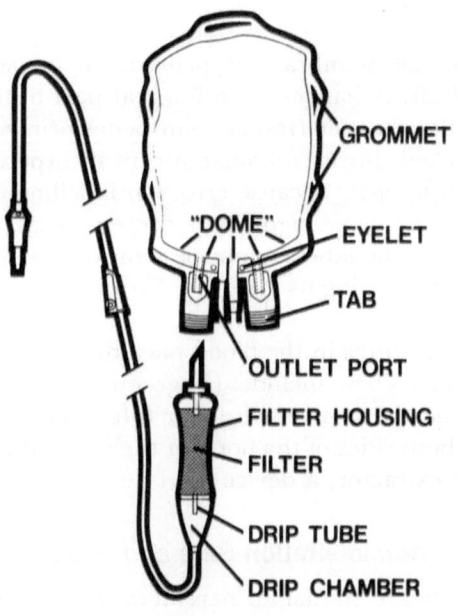

Figure 12.1

There are two outlet ports at the top of each pack in which to insert recipient sets. The sterility of these ports is protected during processing and storage by tabs, two leaves of plastic fused together (Figure 12.2). The port structure remains encased in the sterile 'chamber' formed by the tabs which are separated when the port is to be used. The port itself is similar to those on most plastic fluid containers. There is a tube with a membrane in it, placed high enough so the coupler of the recipient set (blood bankers' language for the spike of the administration set) will be

141

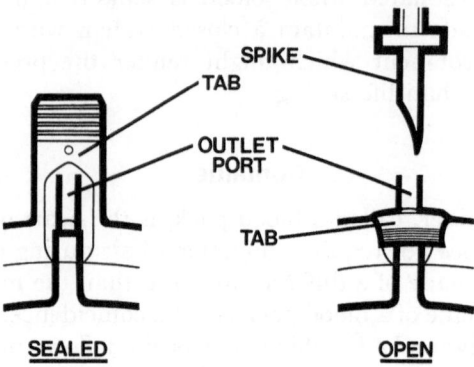

Figure 12.2 The port assembly of a blood collection container remains sterile until opened for use

surrounded when the membrane is penetrated, preventing leakage of blood or entry of air. A hanger is an integral part of the blood pack.

Labels are made of paper (rather than being printed directly on the plastic) and attached during manufacture to incorporate the extensive language required by law. Because errors in labelling or changes made after cross-match can have significant consequences, these labels are 'welded' to the bag. The label cannot be removed by soaking, scraping, or prying without destroying its integrity. No wilful or inadvertent switch can be made.

There are other features in the blood pack design that are not used in its transfusion mode. These include: (1) grommets (slots along each side of the pack) to hold the segmented donor tubing or pilot tubes, and (2) eyelets (holes on both sides of the ports at the top of the bag) to hold the pack in a plasma extractor, a device used during the processing phase.

Administration Sets and Filters

Blood recipient sets are similar to parenteral fluid administration sets. The major parts are the connector (spike), filter housing and drip chamber, tubing and Luer connector. There is no significant difference between the connector of a blood set and the spike of an administration set. (Readers who desire further detail on this point should refer to Chapter 2.)

A filter is mandated by US and UK government regulation for the transfusion of whole blood and components. Its purpose is to capture the 'debris' that accumulates in stored blood, including fibrin strands, platelet and white cell aggregates. The amount of this material in the blood increases with time of storage. The standard filter is made of nylon

142

mesh and has a nominal pore size of 170–200 μ. Its area is about 5 square inches. As debris is captured and prevented from entering the patient, the filter surface may become clogged. When several units are being transfused with the same recipient set, the accumulation of fibrin and aggregates may obstruct a significant portion of the filter surface and reduce the intended flow rate of the transfusion. To obviate this problem in locations where multiple unit transfusions are likely such as operating rooms, recovery rooms and emergency care areas of a hospital, several users select a filter which has the same pore size and an enhanced surface (7.5 square inches).

Recently, interest has risen in non-blood cell particulate of a size less than 200 microns which may pass the standard filter. Some investigators believe this material can induce adverse lung changes and cause a shock syndrome. As a result new filter technology has emerged. One approach has been a modification of recipient sets in which the filter pore size is 80 microns. This filter will capture more material than the standard mesh; it will also occlude more rapidly. If better filtration is desired, a microaggregate filter, described later, should be used.

In a blood recipient set the 'drip chamber' has two parts, the filter housing and the drip chamber. They are made from a single large diameter piece of semi-rigid plastic. The filter housing is above the drip chamber on Fenwal and Travenol sets; Abbott, Cutter, and McGaw manufactured sets have the opposite arrangement. The filter housing and drip chamber cannot be disconnected; they are separated by a heat seal. A drip tube is fixed between them so blood can pass from one to the other. When blood has been filtered by the time it reaches the drip tube, the rate setting is based on drops from the end of the tube over a specified time. The size of the drops varies with the manufacturer so it is important to know the correct multiplier (drops/ml) for the set being used (usually it is stated on the set container). A reason for placing the drip tube below the filter is that this configuration inhibits the entry of air into the blood pack during priming of the set.

Tubing extending from the bottom of the drip chamber to the Luer connector can be of several lengths. Some sets are made with 'Y' sites built into this tubing, presumably to accomodate piggyback infusion of drugs, etc. I do not favor inclusion of the 'Y' site in any blood transfusion set because I think blood is almost a sacrosanct material. 'Y' sites disturb streamlined liquid flow, engender fibrin deposition in the tube lumen, may increase destruction (hemolysis) of red cells and other formed elements, give an opportunity to infuse an incompatible solution, and above all encourage abuse of the set by providing a place for entry without special protection against ingress of contamination. For concomitant solution infusions while blood is running in a set, another vascular

143

access should be used. The blood administration path should remain unblemished.

Some sets have large bore tubing to facilitate increased flow, presuming the lumen size of the exit site (the needle or catheter) is also upgraded. These sets are adapted to high volume, rapid flow transfusions such as may be needed for resuscitation in the emergency room. Flow rates may be increased up to 50% when tubing of a larger diameter is used.

OPERATION OF A TRANSFUSION SYSTEM

In the administration of blood the first action is to verify the identity of the patient and the fact the blood is intended for the identified individual. (Later in this chapter there is a description of a mechanical system that adds to the certainty of giving the correct unit.) There is no substitute for a calm and careful ritual in which the transfusionist demonstrates the pack and the patient are intended for each other. Another individual should be present to verify the correlation and should appreciate this 'second opinion' bears as much responsibility as does the person actually conducting the transfusion. Even in the 'organized chaos' of an emergency, careful identification must be made, for a mistake which results in administering the wrong blood can undo all the life saving measures of a trauma team. There is no excuse for a clerical error involving a blood transfusion. The identification routine typically is unique to each institution. It should be learned and followed carefully.

After the patient/pack correlation is made, the unit is readied for transfusion by attaching a recipient set. Initially the blood pack tabs are opened to expose the port. Then the protector is taken off the administration set connector. With the pack inverted (the ports facing upward), the connector is placed into the port tube and pushed forward with some force and a twisting action until it is seated completely. During this maneuver the membrane in the port tube will be penetrated.

The set is primed by squeezing the bag. Enough blood should be pushed out to fill the filter chamber completely. The unit is returned to the upright position, and a level is established in the drip chamber. This procedure differs from the technique for plastic fluid containers. The blood pack method is intended to cover the filter completely in blood and to avoid retrograde entry of air into the bag. (Recall the primary purpose of the special system design for blood.) After a drip chamber level is set (about half full), the clamp which controls rate of delivery is opened sufficiently to fill the tubing to the Luer connector. Then the unit is ready for transfusion.

An alternate technique involving the use of saline also has achieved some popularity and is conducted as follows. A 'Y' set having two leads is selected instead of a simple recipient set with one lead into the filter chamber. A blood pack is placed on the end of one connector and saline (or any solution compatible with blood) on the other. Priming is accomplished with saline in the same fashion as for blood, making sure the filter chamber and part of the drip chamber are filled before the remainder of the set is primed. A venipuncture is made. Because the saline solution is 'water white', a successful vein entry can be visualized more readily than when blood is in the recipient set tubing. For this reason the 'Y' set technique is gaining converts from straight set devotees. Also, it is permissible to pass some saline through the twin leads from one side of the set into the blood pack in order to dilute packed red cells and make them flow more easily. Available instructions for this procedure should be followed carefully to preserve the integrity of the system. A person performing this transfer for the first time should be assisted by a knowledgeable and trained individual who can demonstrate the necessary art.

Flow of blood is usually regulated by the clamp on the set tubing. Using any of the electro-mechanical pumps with special sets for rate control may be unwise; all have casettes designed for pump efficiency with little attention to prevention of red cell destruction. Only pumps and other flow control devices which will accept standard set tubing should be used in transfusing blood. The blood pack is collapsible; it can be squeezed forcefully to administer the contents rapidly when required by emergent clinical indications, such as uncontrolled hemorrhage or profound hemorrhagic shock. Military services have found this characteristic of blood packs helpful, since the manual external pressure technique can be employed in virtually any situation.

SPECIAL ISSUES AND CONSIDERATIONS

Priming solutions

When mixed with blood, certain solutions, notably 5% dextrose and 5% dextrose with 0.2% saline, will produce destruction of red cells and agglutination of white cells and platelets. The reason is no mystery; the solutions are not isotonic with blood and cause the formed elements, particularly red cells, to shrink in size, become more fragile, and break, releasing free hemoglobin. Solutions of 5% dextrose with 0.4–0.9% saline or 0.9% saline are entirely acceptable. The lower saline concentration should be chosen when there is reason to limit the sodium chloride to be infused. Lactated Ringer's solution is unacceptable for any exposure to blood outside the body because it contains sufficient calcium to initiate the clotting mechanism which is inhibited by an anticoagulant for the purposes of storage and manipulation of the blood. Solutions which commonly are (and are not) used with blood are shown in Tables 12.1 and 12.2.

145

Table 12.1 Solutions NOT recommended for use with transfusions

Solution	Result
5% Dextrose in water	Clumping and hemolysis
5% Dextrose in 0.2% saline	Hemolysis
Lactated Ringer's	Clotting

Table 12.2. Intravenous solutions suggested for use with blood transfusions

5% Dextrose in 0.4% saline
5% Dextrose in 0.9% saline
0.9% Saline
Plasmalyte A pH 7.4

Red cell destruction, clotting and agglutination can occur with even a minimal exposure to contraindicated solutions. Therefore, a 5% dextrose infusion should be followed by several minutes of saline or other compatible fluid before blood is administered through the same set.

Recipient Set Change

Blood transfusion causes accumulation of debris in the filter and other parts of the set. When a sugar containing solution follows blood administration, an ideal medium for the growth of bacteria is established (nitrogen and glucose). A very low level of contamination can propagate rapidly in this environment, resulting in the potential infusion of a 'bacterial culture'. To avoid this risk, the recipient set should be changed upon completion of a blood transfusion if other fluids are to be given thereafter. It is essential to remove nitrogen from the system in order to re-establish the usual low risk of contamination.

Filters

During the last few years there has been interest in the removal of non-physiologic debris by the use of microaggregate filters. These filters have a very large operational surface. Screen and depth filters (and even a combination) are available. Depth filters are a more desirable configuration in my view. Many units of whole blood and packed cells can be transfused through these filters with minimal reduction in desired flow rates and efficiency. There are several products, and before choosing the lowest priced item, it is wise to compare actual, not claimed, performance characteristics.

An unresolved question is when to use these special filters. Since one unit transfusions are medically contraindicated, the issue begins with two units. The real problem is a lack of good, relevant information about the adverse effects of microaggregates. For instance, it not proven they initiate, sustain or synergize adverse circumstances to normal pulmonary function. Several studies have been published, all of which are flawed in some manner so the results cannot be extrapolated directly. I have seen no impressive evidence for a dose response effect where increasing quantities of debris cause incremental physiologic malfunction. Without reliable data whatever policy is established will be based to a considerable extent on theory rather than fact.

A reasonable approach may be that microaggregate filters should be used routinely where multiple unit transfusions are most frequent, in the operating suite and emergency room. While a policy of microaggregate filtering of all blood may be sustainable on the evidence available, there are several issues, including cost effectiveness, which probably will not be settled for some time. When microaggregate filters are employed, they must be removed along with the recipient set assembly immediately after the transfusions are complete. Priming directions must be followed carefully and explicitly for each manufacturer. Filter malfunction will occur if improper procedures are used.

Component Therapy

Packed red cells rather than whole blood are administered except when treating for hemorrhage. The packed red cell preparation is derived from whole blood by centrifuging the blood pack and expressing the plasma carefully into another bag. Red cells remain in the original pack and are handled as whole blood for administration purposes. In this manner more than one recipient can derive benefit from one unit of donor blood, increasing the efficient utilization of a precious natural resource.

Techniques have been developed to isolate and obtain other formed elements of whole blood such as white cells and platelets. The ability to transfuse these delicate structures in sufficient quantity to produce a therapeutic effect has meant that bone marrow suppressive therapy for the treatment of malignant solid tumors and leukemia can be carried into dosages where the chance for cure is enhanced. Other types of bone marrow pathology can also be treated, such as toxic chemical and accidental radiation exposure, and idiopathic thrombocytopenia. Several different mechanical means have been developed to obtain these components without adverse effect on the donor. The separation, storage and transfusion of these components usually requires special apparatus, such as different plastic container formulations and rubber free administration sets. The administration of platelet and white cell packs should follow a specific local protocol which must be observed carefully to gain the greatest benefit for the recipient.

Therapeutic leukopheresis, lymphopheresis, and apheresis are similar techniques recently emerged from the research laboratory. These treatments consist of extracorporeal on line processing of a patient's blood to remove components which are thought to be harmful. The treatment is non-specific at present. Immunologists have an interest, and myasthenia gravis is said by many investigators to benefit from apheresis. Another useful application seems to be the management of acute rejection reactions following kidney transplantation. However, constantly improving immunosuppressive technology may make this treatment outmoded before it becomes proven and popular. It is too early to know if long term adverse effects result for the patient who undergoes several episodes of therapeutic apheresis. More time will be necessary to define the place of this therapy.

Transfusion Reactions

Two aspects of this unhappy event will be discussed: what can be done to prevent it, and what to do when it occurs.

There were 44 fatal hemolytic transfusion reactions reported to the Bureau of Biologics, Food and Drug Administration between 1976 and 1978 inclusive. The source of error was identified in 38 of these reactions.

*7 – Incorrect crossmatch sample or documentation
*17 – Wrong patient received the transfusion
*9 – Administrative error in the hospital laboratory
4 – Technical error in the compatibility test
1 – Incompatible blood transfused before testing was completed.

A majority of transfusion reactions can be traced to a clerical or manipulative error (designated by the asterisk) rather than an incorrect crossmatch in the laboratory. Usually some person takes a shortcut around an established control, either because there is an environment that seems to justify less diligence or because an individual becomes too casual. Every step, obtaining blood from the potential recipient, making crossmatches, and administering the blood product must be performed in a careful manner. There is no substitute for intensity and rigor. If you do not know, if you are unsure, or if there is something which does not fit exactly as expected, **DO NOT** administer the blood until the issue is entirely clear. For instance, do not be pressured by time or alleged urgent need into accepting a unit with a smudged identification just because there is a 'crisis' and someone says they can read the name even if you cannot. Similarly, if there is any question that a specimen for crossmatch may have been mixed up, destroy the tube and obtain another. **DO NOT GUESS!**

In addition to standard procedures for administering the correct blood, there are adjunct techniques I believe worthy of serious consideration, an insurance policy of sorts. The system with which I am most familiar is called Typenex. It consists of a bracelet which is labelled with the patient's name *at the same time* a label is prepared for the crossmatch sample tube (a carbon copy like mechanism is employed). The bracelet has several numbered adhesive tags attached. One is placed on the crossmatch request; the others accompany the crossmatch tube to the laboratory and are detached and placed on acceptable units as testing is completed. When a unit is taken to the recipient's bedside, the usual ritual of patient identification, crossmatch verification and unit matching is performed. The bracelet which has been attached to the patient previously is compared with the number label on the unit. They should be the same because at one time the label was part of the bracelet. In the Typenex system the patient is physically tied to the sample tube when the tube label and bracelet are prepared as a single step. No greater certainty can be achieved. The Typenex system (or any similar methodology) is not intended to replace traditional methods for assuring transfusion of the correct blood product unit, just as an insurance policy should not be the primary prevention for a fire.

A transfusion reaction usually is caused by leukocytes, platelets or plasma proteins, because detection tests for red cell incompatibilities (the other cause of a reaction) are performed before the transfusion is given. Only rarely do these tests fail to uncover an unusual and unexpected red cell related effect (four of the Bu Bio investigated reactions). Symptoms and signs of a transfusion reaction vary in kind and magnitude. Pain in the kidney area, dark urine, nausea and vomiting, shortness of breath, pyrexia and hypotension must be presumed to have a genesis in blood being transfused, unless an alternate cause is quickly apparent and identified with certainty (Table 12.3).

A BLOOD TRANSFUSION SHOULD BE STOPPED AT THE FIRST SIGN OF A REACTION. The unit and attached administration set must be refrigerated and sent to the blood bank as soon as possible. All transfusion reactions must be reported immediately to the attending physician *and* the blood bank. A tube of blood which will clot to produce serum is drawn promptly and sent to the blood bank with a written notice of reaction. A similar specimen should be drawn about 24 hours later and transmitted to the same laboratory. Samples of urine are collected and retained until notice directing disposition is received.

Treatment of the patient consists of enhancing fluid flow through the kidneys, using either furosemide or mannitol. This therapy should be

Table 12.3. Transfusions–Signs, Symptoms, Management

Symptom(s)	Sign(s)	Management
Pruritis	Urticaria	Administer rapid acting antihistamine Observe for further difficulties Notify physician
Anxiety	Flushing	Stop transfusion
Palpitations	Chills	Stop transfusion; maintain intravenous access
Dyspnea	Tachycardia	Stop transfusion; administer rapid acting anthistamine
Headache	Restlessness	See text for sample collection Notify physician
Chest pain	As above	Stop transfusion
Flank or back pain	Red urine	Stop transfusion; maintain intravenous access
Dyspnea	Bleeding (cause unknown)	Treat shock if present
Headache	Hypotension	Administer diuretic See text for sample collection Notify physician

continued for at least 12 hours or until the urine becomes clear if a color change occurred. If renal failure ensues, appropriate therapy is instituted.

The cause of the reaction should be ascertained if possible, and a complete report made part of the patient record for future reference. Thorough study of even minor transfusion reactions is justified by the hope a similar or worse subsequent difficulty for the patient can be avoided.

Sometimes transfusion *associated* reactions occur which are minor in nature, such as the manifestation of hives. These can be managed usually by the administration of an immediate acting antihistamine (Benadryl); long acting, slow onset antihistamines are not reasonable choices. If a patient is a chronic transfusion recipient and has demonstrated the emergence of skin bullae or other minor reactions on more than one occasion, a prophylactic antihistamine dose given just before the transfusion begins may inhibit cosmetic and systemic discomforts.

All transfusion reactions are a proper subject of medical interest and should not be considered casually.

SUMMARY

Blood administration techniques have reached a significant level of sophistication. They provide a life saving and life giving therapy. Few medical treatments have such a profound and dramatic effect. The present system for blood transfusion is closed, tamper proof, and engineered for maximum efficiency in the use of a natural resource. The system is sufficiently flexible to accommodate innovations that continue to enhance the quality of medical care.

References

1. Ryden, S. E. (1976). Compatibility of blood with intravenous solutions. Chapter V. In *Vein to Vein – A Seminar for Phlebotomists and Transfusionists*. American Association of Blood Banks, pp. 72
2. Honig, C. L. and Bove, J. R. (1980). Transfusion association fatalities: review of bureau of biologics reports. *Transfusion*, **20,** 653.
3. *Blood Component Therapy – A Physician's Handbook*. (Washington, DC: American Association of Blood Banks) 1981
4. Conrad, M. E. (1981). *Seminars in Hematology: Transfusion Problems in Hematology*. (New York: Grune and Stratton)
5. Anonymous, (1981). Transfusion disasters. *Lancet*, **2,** 618
6. Walter, C. W. (1956). Department of Plastic Equipment for Blood Bank Use. *Proceedings of Sixth Congress of the International Society of Blood Tranfusion*, Boston, Mass.
7. Walter, C. W., Bellamy, D. and Murphy, W. P. (1955). The mechanical factors responsible for the rapid infusion of blood. *Surg. Gynecol. Obstet.*, **101,** 115

13

Parenteral Nutrition

Any administration of a calorie providing solution via the parenteral route is termed parenteral nutrition. Modern nomenclature, however, has reserved this designation for the technology of giving substantial quantities of carbohydrate calories, protein, and lipid intravenously. TPN (Total Parenteral Nutrition) is a term often used to describe all high osmolality, central vein delivered material. It is a misnomer. Not all parenteral nutrition patients receive nutrition exclusively (totally) by the intravenous route. This designation has been extended further by some to another phrase, partial parenteral nutrition (PPN), meaning a solution of calories and protein delivered into a peripheral vein (as opposed to central vein). The site of delivery has nothing to do with the partial or total nature of the therapy. These classifications are meaningless and confusing. Until a few years ago the word hyperalimentation was applied indiscriminately to nearly everything involving glucose – amino acid solutions. These fluids are only 'hyper' when compared with common solutions.

The proper designations are parenteral alimentation or parenteral nutrition, reserving the modifiers total and partial to indicate the degree of support being given through the vascular route, not the specific blood vessel into which the infusion is being made.

It is my opinion parenteral nutrition is the second of two momentous advances in parenteral therapy in this half of the twentieth century. The first was the development of the closed system which has contributed so impressively to the safe and efficient collection of whole blood and the administration of its components. The adaptation of the closed system to solutions was a corollary triumph which brought significantly better patient care. Now, parenteral nutrition has preserved many lives, and has extended opportunities for care into several areas previously denied

153

to the physician because the patient could not be given adequate support to sustain special treatments.

It is the purpose of this chapter to review technology associated with the use of parenteral nutrition. It will be left to others to discuss the medical science of the treatment.

COMPONENTS OF PARENTERAL NUTRITION

An adequate diet for a normal individual consists of a mixture of carbohydrates, proteins and fat. To simulate normal oral intake, the same components should be present in a parenterally administered diet, although not necessarily in the same relationship to each other. There are different considerations in parenteral formulae which mandate alteration of the typical ratios found in an oral diet of the three substances.

Protein was supplied for parenteral use for many years as a hydrolysate, milk or beef blood treated with acid or enzymes to break up large size proteins and turn them into individual amino acids (about 60% of the formula) or small chains of amino acids called peptides. The beef source material was called a fibrin hydrolysate; the milk source was named casein hydrolysate. The latter was most common worldwide. Although certain advantages in utilization were claimed for fibrin hydrolysate, factually there is no difference between the two sources. Because they make up a large part of the hydrolysate solutions (40%), utilization of peptides is an important consideration. There continue to be differences of opinion about the capability of the human to metabolize peptides.

A few years ago, it became possible to assemble a protein solution from its individual amino acid parts. No peptides were included. Thus, concern for partial availability was obviated. These new solutions, known as crystalline amino acid formulations, have supplanted hydrolysates in many ways. They are advantageous because they can be formulated specifically, giving attention to normalize some physiologic alterations which appear during parenteral nutrition with the naturally sourced hydrolysate. Even though they are more expensive, crystalline amino acid solutions justify the extra cost in their certainty of utilization, special formulation and reliability of structure.

There are many forms of carbohydrate which have been used in parenteral nutrition. The popularity of certain substances is geographic in nature, but there seems to be a worldwide consensus for dextrose over all other available substances. Typical alternates have been maltose, fructose, invert sugar, sorbitol, and xylitol. The last is truly different from the others. Xylitol has been studied with allegedly disastrous consequences in Australia. It has a few advocates in Europe and Japan. It seems acceptable as a non-sugar oral flavoring agent. The true safety of parenterally administered xylitol remains an enigma.

154

Fructose (fruit sugar, levulose) has been used extensively in parenteral solutions. Recent studies have shown its metabolism results in glucose, either directly (70%) or through lactate and then to glucose (30%). It is not true that the metabolism of fructose occurs independent of insulin and that fructose is the carbohydrate of choice for patients having altered glucose metabolism (diabetes mellitus, etc.). Since the immediate breakdown product of fructose is glucose for more than two thirds of the original quantity, insulin is required in substantial amounts. There is danger in believing fructose utilization does not require insulin; the consequences will be failure to recognize or even look for a mounting hyperglycemia.

Invert sugar contains one half dextrose and one half fructose. That portion which is fructose will follow the metabolic pathways noted above. Dextrose will be metabolized in the usual fashion.

Sorbitol is a sugar alcohol and has been favored by some because it can be heated with a protein without the development of a brown color. Therefore, a final parenteral nutrition formulation containing both carbohydrate and protein can be terminally sterilized, imparting to the solution all of the favorable aspects of this process compared to a requirement for post-sterilization admixture when dextrose is the carbohydrate source. Even with these apparent advantages the balance of all considerations is in favor of not using sorbitol for parenteral nutrition. Sorbitol is merely one metabolic step away from fructose; all of it quickly becomes fructose *in vivo*. Also, the disposition of high energy bonds to make conversions from lactate to glucose is too high a metabolic price to pay for the claimed benefits of sorbitol.

There remains only dextrose (Japanese physicians occasionally favor maltose, but its low renal threshold makes it disadvantageous to administer effectively in high concentration). The starting concentration of dextrose used for parenteral nutrition is sometimes as high as 70% and most often 50%. These fluids have a consistency not unlike syrup and are more sensitive to the heat of sterilization than their 5% and 10% counterparts. Therefore, it may be noted from time to time that 50–70% dextrose is not 'water white' but instead seems tinged with yellow. The best information available presently is this quality is cosmetic and not physiologically or pharmacologically adverse. The high concentration of starting material, and even the somewhat lower but nevertheless impressive levels (usually 25–35%) of the final mixture (protein and dextrose), mandate special considerations for the administration of these fluids which will be discussed later.

Another source of energy for parenteral nutrition is fat. It is a necessary element in any parenteral nutrition formula. The advantage of fat is that it provides many calories/gram (10.0 cal/g versus 3.4 cal/g for monohydrate dextrose) in a solution of low osmolality. Therefore, depending on the amount of dextrose in the final mixture, a parenteral nutrition formulation can be made of carbohydrate, fat and protein which may be given by other than central vein catheter. Recent studies of fat as an energy source in acutely ill patients suggest it can be an adequate replacement for all but 150–200 g of dextrose. This fact may facilitate development of a solution which can be tolerated by peripheral veins.

ADMINISTRATION

The major advance which occurred in the late 1960s, making possible the infusion of high calorie content carbohydrate solutions along with protein, was the refinement of the centrally terminated intravenous catheter. This device has been discussed in Chapter 9. Through it solutions having an osmolality intolerable for peripheral veins of small and medium size can be infused into a large vein, such as the vena cava, where substantial blood flow dilutes the formulation immediately.

The dosage for typical central vein parenteral nutrition is 2–4 liters each day. Some physicians prefer to introduce the treatment gradually, giving 1000 ml on the first day and increasing thereafter. Somewhat dissimilar from other infusions, parenteral nutrition fluids are administered throughout the 24 hour day. It is quite important that a fixed rate of infusion be established and maintained to portion the total daily fluid order in an even manner without significant changes in blood glucose levels. For this purpose pumps are used quite often, particularly when low flow rates for neonates are prescribed. For the nurse who finds through some unexpected event the stipulated amount of infusate has not been administered in the prescribed time ('behind' on the fluids – also 'behind' the eight ball), there is a great temptation to increase flow rate temporarily. Such action may change the dextrose balance considerably. Instead, the proper rate should be established, and the previous fault made known in the nurses' report of the patient chart with the expectation an understanding physician will be tolerant. Anyone who does not appreciate these problems can occur has little experience in patient care. Of course, repeated occurrences must be given proper corrective attention.

Intravenous lipid is given through an administration set arrangement which has a Y site near the needle adapter, providing a short route into the vein. Another option is to mix the lipid directly with the dextrose and amino acid solutions. Physical incompatability of the lipid, dextrose and amino acid mixture is not the problem originally perceived if the solution is made correctly.

Amino acid/carbohydrate/lipid solutions generally can be delivered into the peripheral vein if the total osmolality is below 800/mosm/kg. Even at that level some patients will complain of burning at the infusion site.

For several years it was claimed i.v. fat facilitated the peripheral administration of high osmolality solutions by 'coating the vein wall' (This concept reminds me of the theory that drinking milk or eating butter before an alcoholic binge ameliorates the effect of alcohol on gastric mucosa and the central nervous system by coating the stomach – remember those days?) Actually the benefit of i.v. fat is in its dilutional effect. Its osmolality is about 300 mosm/kg when it contains glycerol. When mixed with a 1000–1500 mosm/kg solution, the latter level will be reduced, depending on the ratio of the mixtures. This downward change may not be enough, resulting in irritation at the infusion site and proximally in the vein course. Changing the infusion site every 24 hours would be important in treating these patients.

There are a few physicians who advocate the exclusive use of amino acid solution with no carbohydrate or fat. This fluid can be given in a peripheral vein almost without exception. However, the practice has lost considerable popularity and is physiologically without merit. A base of 150–200 g of dextrose must be included to achieve adequate protein sparing. Minimizing the dextrose or eliminating part of the parenteral nutrition formulation occasionally is justified by the absolute need for peripheral vs. central vein administration.

COMPLICATIONS

There are several complications which may accompany parenteral nutrition. Some are medical (hyperglycemia, hyperosmotic coma, etc.); others are related to technique.

The most feared problem ensuing from parenteral nutrition therapy is septicemia. Infection is believed to stem from poor technique in preparing and handling the solution and catheter. There continues to be much debate about whether the infection originates externally and travels down the catheter course to the vein or 'implants' on the catheter from micro-organisms in the bloodstream. There are significant reductions in the incidence of septicemia when a hospital standardizes the management of these solutions and devices. I have commented already on the features of closed system containers, an externally applied pump mechanism, and the non-irritating silicone catheter, central or peripheral. Together these make up a good system when they are assembled by knowledgeable, concerned, attentive pharmacy and nursing personnel. An immutable institution protocol is a must for successful parenteral nutrition. The specific content of the protocol actually is not so important as its existence; it should be followed rigorously by all personnel, and its inception should represent the combined thinking of medical, nursing and pharmacy staffs.

Occasionally, I have found a protocol which includes an unusual or complex maneuver inserted shortly after recognition of a single adverse patient reaction. These steps frequently benefit neither the patient nor the protocol. They may introduce an alternate, unrecognized danger. Don't overreact!

A good parenteral nutrition catheter care protocol exemplifies sound judgment in selecting equipment, supplies and suitable procedures. Above all, it is uncomplicated. An example is presented in the appendix.

IDEAL METHODOLOGY

I believe the ideal way to handle parenteral nutrition in any hospital is to assign responsibility to a team (Figure 13.1). Whether it has a strong

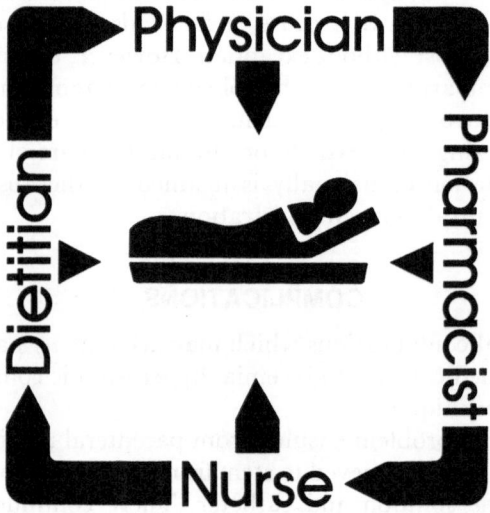

Figure 13.1 This symbol exemplifies the team approach to parenteral nutrition

consultative or an actual control role is immaterial. If it performs effectively, the team will be appreciated and its continuing existence assured. The team should consist of a physician, a pharmacist, a nurse and a dietitian. Each has specific responsibilities as shown in the accompanying table (Table 13.1). Each member should be the communication

Table 13.1

Elements in parenteral nutrition therapy	Primary responsibility
1. Indications, patient selection, therapy direction	Physician
2. Solution formulation, protection, quality control	Pharmacist
3. Administration, patient monitoring	Nurse
4. Conversion to enteral feeding, formulation monitoring	Dietitian

link between the team and his/her colleagues. In the best circumstance the team (or individual members) visits the bedside of each patient receiving nutrition support, parenteral or oral, on a daily basis. The value of such attention becomes obvious in improved results and avoided complications.

All of the supplies for parenteral nutrition should be intended for single use (disposable). Only the pump which is discussed later in this chapter and more extensively in Chapter 8 is permanent.

As noted previously in the review of admixture procedures (Chapter 6), combining the various components of the parenteral nutrition prescription (amino acids, glucose, lipid, electrolytes, vitamins and trace elements) is the proper responsibility of a pharmacist who works in a controlled environment for such procedures and benefits from a well designed quality control program. (Closed systems that allow for mixing of components outside of a laminar flow controlled environment are on the horizon.)

The final mixture should be placed in a closed container which is the most certain way to prevent ingress of contaminants during transit and storage before the solution reaches the patient. A special unit has been designed to accommodate the unique requirements of parenteral nutrition (Figure 13.2). It is an empty, flexible plastic container with an attached set having a bifurcation ending in spikes that fit conveniently into the amino acid, glucose and lipid source units. Other additives are made through the port which is covered by the rubber stopper. At the completion of the admixture procedure the unit, properly labeled, should be refrigerated to inhibit growth of any contaminating organisms which may have slipped into the solution in spite of due care. A temperature of about 4°C should be maintained until just before use. The relatively slow transit time of liquid through the administration set lumen commonly permits sufficient rewarming to occur (except for the first 50–100 ml) before the solution reaches the patient. If there is concern about this point, the container can be removed from refrigeration 1–2 hours before expected use without fear of adverse consequences. It is not good practice to have the pharmacist attach the administration set. Such an arrangement makes subsequent handling more difficult. It has been demonstrated this connection can be made with a very low risk of contamination in and around the usual nursing station. The addition of admixtures incrementally raises the danger for introduction of micro-organisms into the solution. Manipulation of the administration set contributes almost nothing to this risk.

At many other points in this book I have emphasized the advantages of a truly closed administration system. Nowhere is the concept more important than in parenteral nutrition. The propensity for proliferation of bacteria and fungi in a solution of amino acids and glucose mandates

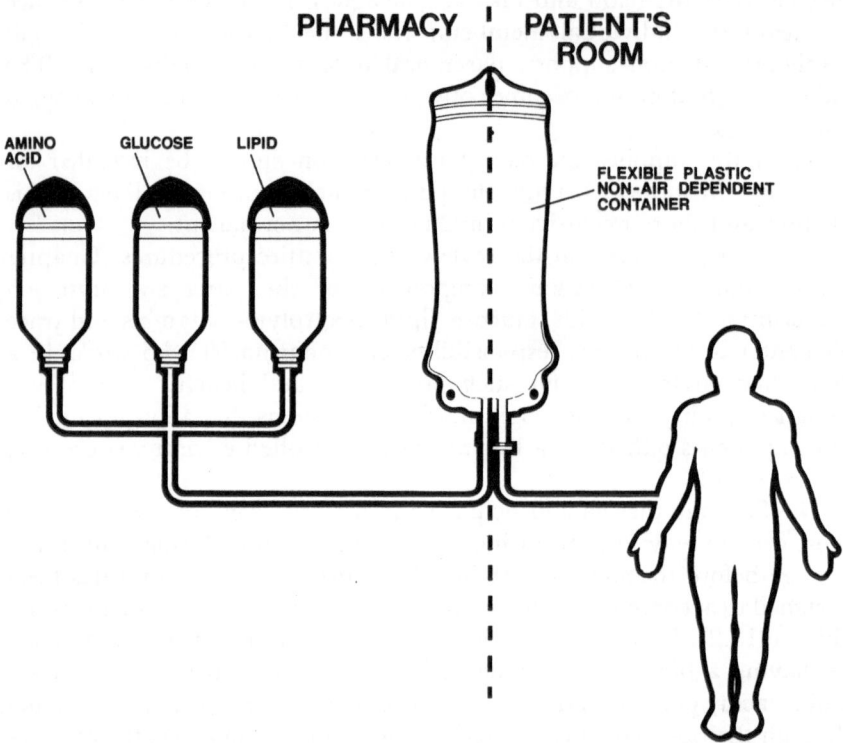

PHARMACY | PATIENT'S
ROOM

AMINO
ACID   GLUCOSE   LIPID

FLEXIBLE PLASTIC
NON-AIR DEPENDENT
CONTAINER

Figure 13.2   The 3 in 1 container (on the right) provides the convenience of a one container system, the safety of central admixture, and non air dependent administration

the ultimate in protection, which should begin before the different liquids are placed in the final container and conclude when the final milliliter has been infused. Nothing less is acceptable.

PATIENT MONITORING

There are several observations which nurses should make routinely of patients receiving parenteral nutrition. This attention can be divided into two categories, mechanical and physiologic.

The nurse is responsible for setting and maintaining proper and constant flow rates of solution as ordered by the physician. Problems relating to flow control have been mentioned already.

Some physicians believe a sudden cessation of parenteral nutrition solution infusion will produce a 'reactive hypoglycemia' because there is insufficient glucose to offset the unrelenting endogenous flow of insulin from a 'stimulated' pancreas. This potential complication has been investigated using continuous blood glucose monitoring equipment. No reactive hypoglycemia was observed in several patients who were tested by suddenly stopping a parenteral nutrition infusion. The hospital protocol should address the correct manner for handling this problem if it occurs during the treatment of a patient. An abrupt accidental stop is *not* a clinical crisis.

Another duty of the nurse is to monitor urine for glucose, and to respond in accordance with protocol stipulations.

The nurse or physician house officer often is the first to see one or more of the several physiologic signs of potential danger. Patient temperature is important; it can be the initial sign of infection, which when suspected should initiate a series of actions to diagnose the cause and alleviate the problem immediately. In Chapter 9 proper catheter care and monitoring for difficulties relating to these devices are discussed. Other vital signs (pulse, respiration) can indicate cardiorespiratory failure which may relate to the amount of fluid being infused. Careful intake and output records are not just a mechanical routine; they are an important measure of overall fluid balance.

There comes a time in the management of nearly every patient when transition to an oral route of nutrition (eating) is indicated. Sometimes, this stage is not anticipated enthusiastically by the patient who may continue to have the mental perception of serious illness and no fully developed desire to accelerate recovery. It is at this time the professional skills of the nurse and dietitian are tested most severely. Together they must guarantee the patient receives encouragement, attractive food within prescribed limits, and parenteral supplementation to make up for energy not being taken orally. The balancing act between oral and parenteral alimentation is a daily duty and a cooperative adventure.

As the patient moves into the phase of full oral support, the dietitian becomes the dominant team member, responsible for maintaining the quality and quantity of food intake.

EXPECTED RESULTS

The goal of parenteral nutrition is to achieve positive nitrogen balance for those patients suffering from malnutrition, whatever the cause. In some instances the therapy is anticipatory, ordered by the physician when extended periods of no oral energy intake are typical of the patient's illness or treatment being given. Parenteral nutrition can provide a major assistance to the patient seeking to regain strength and health. It can be administered with minimal complications, making the risk/benefit to the patient quite attractive.

SUMMARY

Parenteral nutrition is intended to help restore/maintain nitrogen equilibrium and support total energy balance. It must be administered with minimal complications for the patient and few difficulties for the staff. It is not unusually complex or dangerous if careful attention to detail is exercised. Because parenteral nutrition has unique aspects that involve several different health care disciplines, a team approach works effectively. Members of the team should not be so dominant that their work results in abrogation of duties by others. Instead, a properly functioning team serves as a focal point for improving therapy and gives assistance in the form of instruction and memory stimulation to those having direct responsibility for individual patient care.

Parenteral nutrition should be available at every hospital. A hospital staff can be organized to handle most treatments properly within the reasonable limits of its resources.

Bibliography

1. Byrne, W. J., Lippe, B. M., Strobel, C. T. *et al.* (1981). Adaptation to increasing loads of total parenteral nutrition: metabolic, endocrine and insulin receptor responses. *Gastroenterology*, **80**, 947
2. Anonymous. (1981). Hyperalimentation standards of practice. *Oncology Nursing Forum*, **8**, 36
3. Powell-Tuck, J., Lennard-Jones, J. E., Lowes, J. A. *et al.* (1979). Intravenous feeding in a gastroenterological unit. *J. Clin. Pathol.*, **32**, 549
4. Ashcraft, K. W. and Leape, L. L. (1970). Candida sepsis complicating parenteral feeding. *J. Am. Med. Assoc.*, **212**, 454
5. Ausman, R. K. and Hardy, G. (1978). Metabolic complications of parenteral nutrition. In *Advances in Parenteral Nutrition*, pp. 403-410. (Lancaster: MTP)
6. Ausman, R. K., Quebbeman, E. J. and Altmann, C. L. (1983). Liver malfunction associated with parenteral nutrition. In *Advances in Clinical Nutrition*, pp. 303-312. (Lancaster: MTP)
7. Quebbeman, E. J., Ausman, R. K. and Schneider, T. C. (1982). A Re-evaluation of energy expenditure during parenteral nutrition. *Ann. Surg.*, **195**, 282
8. Elman, R. (1948). *Parenteral Alimentation in Surgery*. (New York: Paul B. Heober)

14

Irrigating Solutions

USES

Irrigating solutions differ primarily from typical intravenous fluids in the way they are packaged. There are formulations which are suitable exclusively for external application while others may be used for bathing or washing body cavities which have a direct access to the vascular system. There are some irrigating solutions which can be adapted for any mode.

Specific examples of each group are easy to identify. Products prepared to accomplish antisepsis, essentially all of which are applied topically with great care to avoid stipulated sensitive tissues, fall into one category. Solutions for bladder irrigation, including plain water (water without solutes) are in another group. These formulations may be marginally compatible with blood and/or are toxic to certain organs or tissues which are distant to the site of application. Some solutions which are infused intravenously or intra-arterially can be used for irrigation applications as well (e.g. saline).

Other common uses in addition to direct patient contact include removal of lubricant powder from sterile gloves, filling of containers which require a liquid reservoir for proper function (O_2 humidifiers) and rinsing of sterilized instruments before use. Applications of irrigating solutions seem limited only by the imagination of the manipulator.

This liberal framework of usage dictates that certain quality standards be met or exceeded so irrigating fluids do not become dangerous to the patient. Given the possibility an irrigating solution can become an unplanned intravenous solution, irrigants should receive the same care and attention in manufacture and use as products intended for parenteral administration. In some hospitals where in-house manufacture of intravenous solutions has been terminated in favor of commercial purchase, preparation of irrigating solutions was permitted to continue, even though available processing equipment was old, supplies of 'reusable' glass containers were difficult to obtain and demanded increasing maintenance expenditure, or the staff recognized certain mandatory control procedures were too complex to implement. To retain some of the monetary advantages usually attributed to local preparation of solutions, the old equipment and techniques were diverted to making irrigating fluids in the mistaken and misguided belief that less critical applications such as wound irrigation do not require quality at the level of intravenous injections. 'After all' it was said, 'the wound is contaminated already', thereby dismissing the need for concern and admitting the possibility of non-sterility in some units. This kind of thinking is reprehensible and irresponsible. Informed practitioners will greet such expressions with disdain and concern.

If a manufacturing system and its products are unsuitable for intravenous use, they are unsuitable for an application which includes a need for sterile fluids. Any compromise with this position will harm some patient ultimately.

There is no justification for local manufacture of parenteral or irrigation fluids.

TYPES OF CONTAINERS

As in parenteral fluids the two types of container materials used for irrigating solutions are glass and plastic. All of the containers are rigid or semi-rigid; all are air-dependent, that is they require that air be admitted to replace the simultaneous exit of liquid. Thus, all are 'open' systems.

Glass containers generally are of two subtypes, distinguished primarily by different methods to seal the bottle. The variety commonly used for local solution manufacture is a round flask with a neck opening surrounded and crowned by a large rubber donut. After the bottle has been filled and placed in the sterilizer, a plastic dome is fitted loosely on top of the donut allowing for the ingress and egress of air so that pressures can equalize as the sterilizer temperature and fluid temperature move upward in the same direction (but at a different rate). When the heat cycle is completed, the sterilizer is opened, and as soon as possible the plastic dome is pressed firmly into position in the rubber donut. Further cooling thereafter causes an increase in the air space in the container, now theoretically sealed from communication with the external environment. No makeup air is available; a negative pressure develops. Before the unit is opened, the user is expected to strike the bottom of the container with the heel of the hand, trying to detect a sharp click which indicates the presence of a vacuum and presumptively confirms the unit has remained sealed since heat treatment. Unfortunately, this very attractive theory is somewhat oversimplified for common practice. Its most obvious fault is that not everyone checks for the presence of a vacuum before placing the unit in use. Also, the 'click-check' is not completely reliable. Small leaks may be insufficient to relieve all the vacuum and will go undetected (false 'click check').

The most serious flaw in this container system is its mandatory re-use (cost dictates it cannot be discarded). After each sterilization the rubber becomes more brittle and deteriorated, leading to poor fitting of plastic domes. In my opinion, there is no redeeming feature which justifies the use of such a system. Fortunately, it is increasingly difficult to obtain these glass, rubber and plastic parts so that few hospitals will employ this system in the future.

The alternative glass system which is supplied commercially is being rapidly supplanted by plastic units which are described later in this chapter. The glass bottle has a classic shape (if it can be said that any glass container is classic). Its overall circumferential dimension and height are dictated by the quantity of fluid contained. Those of a size greater than one liter are quite heavy and cumbersome. The exposed surface of the neck is molded into threads when the bottle is made. The cap is usually metal and has a rubber washer or gasket to form the seal between the top of the bottle and the inside of the cap. It is not expected the container or cap will be used more than once, although there are some hospitals in which at least the glass is recovered from nursing stations and recycled. Occasionally, even the caps are treated in the same manner. Only the most foolish could believe in the safety of such a practice in which an effort is made to reduce overall costs at a considerable risk to the patient and medical care personnel.

In the last few years study and innovation have been motivated by clinical incidents in the United States which brought some shortcomings of the above screw cap closure into focus. Recognizing the basic advantages of a plastic container in terms of diminished weight and fragility, a square (sometimes rectangular) design has been developed with a modified screw cap closure intended specifically to sustain thread sterility up to the immediate time of use. Each manufacturer has made a slightly different product. This advance has been at the cost of a minimal increase in price which is quite justified for the benefits delivered. The basic theory is that there are two sealing surfaces between the cap and container. One is in the typical location between the top of the plastic bottle and the gasket inside of the cap. The second usually is lower on the cap where it and the bottle are designed in such a manner they can be sealed together. In the most adequate exemplification of this design, the second seal is independent of and ruptured before the primary seal.

165

DESIRABLE SYSTEM FEATURES

There are several key features which should be part of any irrigating solution system selected.

(1) The container must have a tamper proof seal. It must be evident immediately the unit has been opened previously so that it is not used again.

(2) The container should have a large neck (about 40 mm). Smaller orifices admit air poorly during pouring, and there is much gurgling and bubbling as the water flows out in direct conflict with the air entering to take its place. Splashing can lead to uncontrolled pouring and contamination.

(3) The product should be available in several sizes so the temptation for a second use is minimized by selecting the appropriate quantity for a given application.

Problems mentioned above allow for the possibility of fluid contamination sometime before use. There is another event of different but equal importance – contamination during use. The thread tracks on the bottle neck and metal cap can provide a path for micro-organisms to extend to the upper portions of the closure. If the thread area is not maintained organism free, contaminants are drawn up as the cap is removed and deposited on the lip of the glass where they will be washed into the solution or backward into the container. A common practice of irrigating solution users is to pour from the container only the amount intended for immediate use and then replace the cap which may have been deposited on a non-sterile work surface or touch contaminated during removal and manipulation. The next time the cap is taken off, microbes will pass from the cap to the bottle to the solution. Contaminated threads can lead to a contaminated solution. Exercise great care in re-using the container to avoid these difficulties. *Never use a bottle for different patients. Never retain a previously opened irrigating container for more than 12 hours.*

Because the water or saline in irrigating containers is of the same quality (when made commercially) as for intravascular infusion, there is often a temptation to use the solution as a diluent for lyophilized or crystalline medications. As it is difficult to withdraw the liquid from any pouring container without a significant risk of transgressing its sterility, this practice should be avoided. There are fluid containers specifically designed for the purpose which should be employed for these needs.

SUMMARY

Four important concepts govern the selection and use of irrigating solutions.

166

(1) Do not compromise quality. Irrigating fluid should have the same high attributes as parenteral fluid.

(2) The irrigating container and solution should be used only as indicated on the label. To do otherwise invites problems of several types, the most important of which is contamination.

(3) After irrigating never store partially used solutions. Whatever may be saved will never offset the disadvantages to the patient.

(4) Safety for the user and the patient dictates the selection of plastic containers over glass bottles.

15

New Technologies

The opening chapter of this book described several historical events which were notable in the evolution of intravascular infusions. This chapter provides an insight into emerging technologies which are appearing in hospitals either as new methods of care or major modifications of established techniques, in a sense the opposite end of the spectrum. Included are the following:

(1) Continuous intra-arterial infusion – antitumor chemotherapy
   (a) – short term inpatient
   (b) – long term outpatient,

(2) Continuous intravenous infusion – antitumor chemotherapy
   (a) – long term ambulatory,

(3) Continuous subcutaneous insulin infusion, and

(4) Controlled intermittent infusion.

INTRA-ARTERIAL INFUSION (AMBULATORY)

The purpose of infusing a drug into an artery is to provide direct treatment to a specific anatomical area with a minimally diluted (high concentration) therapeutic agent. Because an artery conducts blood *to* the tissue, a drug placed in the vessel can be expected to 'see' the target immediately (presuming placement close to the organ). The drug is diluted only in flowing blood which passes the catheter during the infusion. The dose delivered to the target is higher than when the same quantity is administered intravenously, presuming some fixation to tissue or metabolism occurs in the target tissue.

Another benefit, in some instances, is that the drug is detoxified by the target organ before it enters the venous circulation and is spread throughout the body. On occasion this detoxification is thought to reduce

169

systemic adverse effects in comparison to intravenous infusion of the same dose.

There are two time frames typically for intra-arterial infusion, intermittent and continuous. The intermittent mode usually is executed by occasional (does not mean haphazard) injections into an artery which is easily accessible by means of a percutaneous puncture. A syringe is the common device used, and the volume administered usually does not exceed 20 ml. The duration of the infusion in nearly every instance is less than 15 minutes; often it is as rapid as 1–2 minutes. The needle is removed immediately after completion of the injection. There are only a few examples of this type of treatment extant today. In years past it has been employed for femoral artery injection of medicine intended to achieve peripheral capillary vasodilation (intractable skin ulcer caused by inadequate arterial blood supply). An example of a single instance intra-arterial infusion is the outmoded transcutaneous insertion of a needle in the common carotid artery to inject a radio-opaque contrast medium for visualization of the arterial supply to the brain, a diagnostic procedure. This less than satisfactory approach has been supplanted by a catheter inserted in a femoral artery and threaded to the location of the aortic arch. The contrast medium is injected after careful positioning of the catheter tip at the orifice of each common carotid artery.

Intermittent infusion provides no distinct advantage unless the drug being administered is fixed to tissue very rapidly followed by a drug/tissue interaction that is favorable to the patient. An example would be the anti-tumor drug nitrogen mustard (HN_2, Mustargen). This agent binds to the first exposed tissue immediately and tightly. It effects an alkylating action promptly, but some drug escapes to spread generally throughout the body. Nitrogen mustard has been supplanted by less toxic agents for the treatment of most tumors, and its intra-arterial use is all but extinct, at least for the present. The intermittent form of intra-arterial drug administration requires no special understanding or treatment technique to sustain its use other than a sound knowledge of anatomy and skill in the manipulation of a needle and syringe. It has been presented to provide a contrast to continuous intra-arterial infusion which is described later.

Renewing the infused drug supply by continuous infusion creates an environment in which there is a constant exposure of tissue to the drug. There may be some fixation to the anatomical area of initial contact, but more likely the effect achieved is one in which the immediate environment of target cells is bathed at all times with the therapeutic agent. Concentration of the drug at this tissue *theoretically* is higher than elsewhere in the body.

The technology of successful continuous intra-arterial infusion requires a catheter to be placed and remain in the artery. Substantial differences between artery and vein mandate that intra-arterial catheters be managed in a different way than their intravenous counterparts.

The insertion of an intra-arterial catheter is accomplished most advantageously during a surgical procedure where the best locations for penetration of the artery and anchoring the catheter can be identified and used. For instance, if during a laparotomy it is judged likely that vascular access to the hepatic artery would be desirable in the post-operative period (to infuse an anti-tumor agent for treatment of a primary or secondary liver tumor), the surgeon may place a catheter by cannulating a branch of the common hepatic artery. The catheter tip ultimately will be located in its ideal position, and the catheter itself will be anchored with non-absorbing sutures at various locations in the abdomen, exiting through a small incision in the skin. Through this device the infusion will be initiated and continued.

Sometimes there is no possible surgical procedure which provides ideal access. Then the ingenuity of the physician is tested, and the co-operative efforts of an entire health care team are put in motion. For instance, a catheter tip in the common hepatic artery might be placed by making an insertion through the skin into the brachial artery, passing the catheter centrally (counter to arterial flow) until reaching the aorta, and then turning it downward (in the direction of arterial flow) until reaching the celiac axis. At that point the tip is pushed forward into the hepatic artery. The reader can visualize at least two acute changes in direction (into the celiac axis and then into the hepatic artery) and one more gradual turn (brachial to descending aorta) (Figure 15.1). It is obvious a radiologist with skill and experience is necessary to do this work. Once placed, the work is not done. A means of securing the catheter at a location in the upper arm considerably distant from the tip must be found so there is adequate protection against infection, suitable arm mobility in order not to impair the patient significantly, and stable positioning of the catheter at all times. Physicians and nurses work together to develop training of the patient to understand what has been done and to care for the catheter. Connections in the tubing system between the catheter and the infusion reservoir (including the pump) *must* be of the Luer lock type. Slip lock or friction lock mechanisms are unacceptable as there is a constant danger of inadvertent disconnection. The system should have a clamp which can be operated simply and easily with one hand immediately adjacent to the first connection between catheter and tubing set. Its purpose is to suspend flow quickly if an accident occurs.

When the system is 'installed' as described and equipped with one of the pumps noted below, it is feasible for the patient to ambulate freely. I have attended such patients who maintained an essentially normal life style (sometimes so normal it appeared even casual). The benefit to the

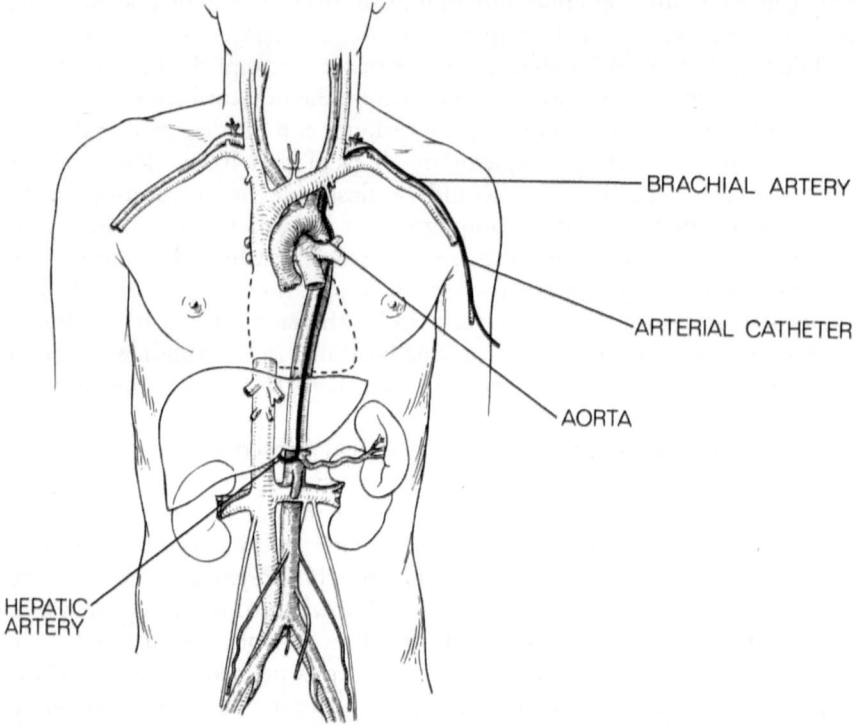

BRACHIAL ARTERY

ARTERIAL CATHETER

AORTA

HEPATIC
ARTERY

Figure 15.1   Route of an intra-arterial hepatic artery catheter inserted from the brachial artery

patient when this degree of freedom from encumbering treatment can be granted is obvious. The quality of life is a joy to behold for all those who make it possible; physicians, nurses, pharmacists and other allied health personnel. Unfortunately, there are several recent reports of morbidity related to intra-arterial catheter placement when it is used for anti-tumor agents such as 5-fluorouracil. Coupled with increasing evidence the intravenous route is equally beneficial, these papers may diminish enthusiasm for intra-arterial treatment.

Intra-arterial infusion is used most frequently for the administration of anti-cancer agents where the tumor is limited to a specific anatomical area served by an identifiable arterial supply. Because many tumors metastasize to the liver where they disrupt vital function, and because major portions of the liver often cannot be resected surgically or treated well with radiotherapy, the hepatic artery has become an increasingly interesting conduit for infusion of drugs like 5-fluorouracil. Another claimed advantage of this treatment modality is that the liver detoxifies some of the drug, thereby limiting the amount of systemic toxicity and increasing the total amount of drug which can be given. Although the liver is an organ with a dual blood supply, it has been shown the artery supplies metastatic growths which push aside and distort the venous structure.

Using a similar theory, tumors of the head and neck region have been treated with infusion of the external carotid artery. Interest in the technique has waxed and waned with the introduction at various times of new anti-tumor agents which seem uniquely suitable for intra-arterial infusion. For this anatomical region the catheter is placed during a surgical procedure in almost all instances. One investigator has reported treating chest wall cutaneous recurrence of a breast tumor through the internal mammary artery. This technique is a sign of ingenuity that will be domonstrated by physicians now that the technique of intravascular infusion has been facilitated with proper equipment and supplies.

There are three major classes of complications associated with intra-arterial infusion: (1) vascular, (2) catheter related, and (3) general. Vascular complications are typical of problems which arise when a foreign body has penetrated into and resides in a vessel, with particular emphasis on the high pressure, arterial part of the vascular tree. Several plastic catheters are quite stiff. The tip may become impinged at a specific site on the artery wall. If the catheter has been fixed to the skin surface on a portion of the anatomy that moves regularly, such as the arm, certain motions may produce a piston effect and cause the tip to penetrate the artery wall. Actually, this complication is made less likely by many turns and bends in the catheter path which take up the pistoning motion rather than transmitting it. When penetration occurs, it is not followed in every instance by a disastrous hemorrhage. Sometimes the catheter plugs the hole nicely, and the real complication is the infusion of medication and fluid outside the vascular space. Depending on location, this phenomenon may go undetected several days during which the drug is not reaching the intended tissues. Of course, there are circumstances in which hemorrhage is the result of penetration. Because the tip location is deep in the body in many instances, often there is little to be done. The patient may be found *in extremis* with almost no time to undertake life saving measures.

The presence of a foreign material in an artery can initiate the clotting cascade with thrombosis as the final result. For some locations and diseases occlusion of the vessel by this means may enhance the therapeutic benefit (such as thrombosis of the hepatic artery). In other instances there is a less happy result. A few physicians prefer to establish some degree of anticoagulation during the infusion, but most afficionados of prolonged intra-arterial treatments have not been troubled sufficiently to justify this step which has its own undesirable effects.

Rarely it has been reported that somehow a catheter is separated from

173

its connector or becomes torn asunder (usually quite mysteriously) so a catheter fragment migrates with the blood flow and embolizes into an area where the vascular lumen is too small to allow further transit. Because many catheters are made of material which may cause a fibrotic reaction or other adverse effect, physicians often have recommended the fragment be removed, even when major surgery is necessary to do so. Frequently, the fragment can be retrieved by employing a second catheter with a loop or other grasping device guided by X-ray visualization.

From time to time a portion of the infusion system outside the body may be severed accidentally by a sharp object. The patient can handle this misadventure quickly by closing the clamp which should always be near the entry of the catheter into the skin. Another approach is to use a connecting tube with a one way valve so that any interruption in the continuity of the tube does not result in back flow of blood. Disconnections have been mentioned previously. They must be obviated prospectively by using Luer lock connections at all sites where parts of the tubing system are joined.

The problem of infection is as real in an intra-arterial infusion as for any location. Special care and attention must be given to any catheter or infusion system manipulations. Changes in the drug reservoir should be made carefully. Skin surface treatment follows the pattern suitable for any percutaneous vascular penetration. When infection occurs, it is often difficult to face the prospect of removing the catheter. If a reasonable search for another cause fails to reveal anything, the choice becomes a decision; the catheter is taken out. Only very rarely is antibiotic treatment successful in controlling and eradicating a catheter fed infectious process without removing the catheter. The benefit of attempting to do so almost always is insufficiently attractive to sustain the risk of proliferation of the infection.

The propulsion of fluid into an artery requires a substantially higher pressure than for venous infusion. Although the arterial intravascular pressure usually does not exceed 200 mmHg, a safe level at which to conduct an intra-arterial infusion is approximately 250 mmHg. The flow need not be pulsatile as there is no indication that simulation of the normal arterial pressure curve provides better penetration of the drug into the tissue. However, constant flow must be sustained.

Many already available infusion pumps serve quite well for the purpose of intra-arterial infusion (*see* Chapter 8). Only those which are occlusive are suitable. A pump that does not embody a design which prevents backflow of fluid at any pressure should not be used. In essentially every instance when this feature is present, the design also provides enough power to give the necessary 250 mmHg propulsive force to the fluid.

Inevitably when pumps are discussed, the twin issues of accuracy

174

and precision surface. For the purpose of infusions (intra-arterial or intravenous) exemplified in the uses cited below, accuracies in the range of ±10% of nominal setting usually are acceptable. Many manufacturers claim much better performance, but often the data proferred in support of the claim have been obtained under ideal conditions which are not seen in a typical clinical setting. Reliability and simplicity are more important attributes than special magnitudes of accuracy. Precision also is important. The flow created by the pump should not change significantly over several hours (even days since some infusions are intended to run for several days). The permissible variation between periods of several hours is approximately ±5% from the initial setting. Minute to minute or even hour to hour changes have little significance, as long as they do not result in wide swings in actual rate of fluid delivery.

Another means of infusing fluid through an artery is provided by applying a constant external pressure to a flexible plastic container such as a 500 ml or 1000 ml Viaflex unit which has the proper concentration of medication added to it. There are sleeves available commercially that incorporate a pneumatic cuff (Figure 15.2). The fluid container is put in

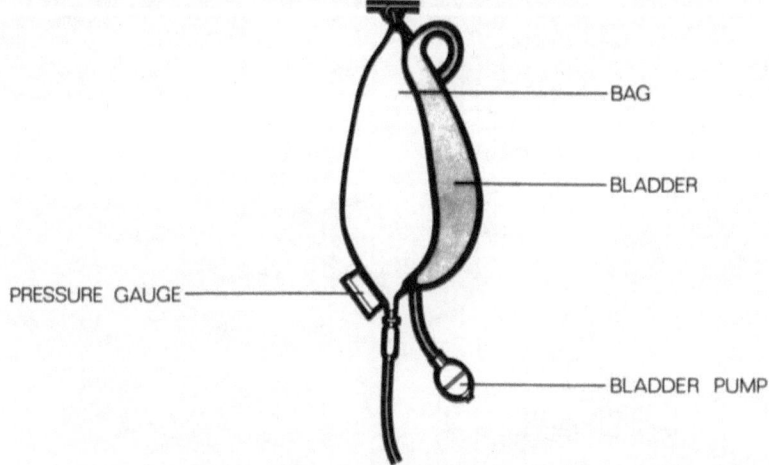

Figure 15.2 The air bladder is filled to the operating pressure, forcing fluid out of the bag which is constrained by a net attached to the air bladder

the sleeve, and a pressure is created by inflating the cuff. Some sense of flow control is achieved by maintaining the pressure in a specified range (usually shown by a green mark on a simple pressure gauge incorporated into the apparatus). The presumption is that if pressure is constant and downstream resistance created by the needle or catheter remains the same, the flow will be constant. Of course, the reader can sense immediately that as the container empties, more pneumatic pressure must be applied. Since emptying is a continuum, and replenishing pressure is an intermittent event related in part to the amount of attention given to the infusion, there will be rather wide variations in flow rate. If not managed properly, flow can stop completely at times, resulting in potential problems of catheter management and difficulty in sustaining a proper concentration of drug in the bloodstream and target tissue. Although it is easy to imagine how a better system for applying pressure continuously and automatically might be devised to improve this situation, there is little impetus to do so because of other disadvantages, such as the amount of fluid which must be given daily and the restriction to full ambulation of the patient because the cumbersome apparatus must be on a tether.

There has evolved a class of pumps which are small in size, capable of delivering minimal amounts of fluid per day, driven by battery power sources that sustain operation over 24–48 hours before recharging is necessary. The rotary peristaltic pump is the best example of such a device. A unit in which I had some hand in the design is shown in Figure 15.3. Fluid propulsion results from the constant motion of a wheel inside

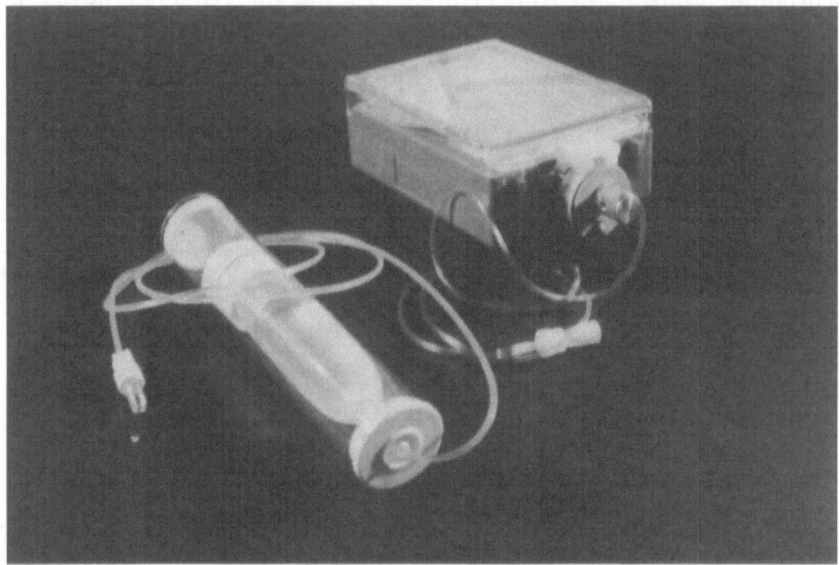

Figure 15.3 Two devices for continuous ambulatory infusion. Upper right–small rotary pump with battery energy source (Travenol MVP). Lower left–Travenol Infusor (see text)

a cage (rotor and jaws). There is a contact point between these parts so the fluid filled tube is squeezed in a manner that milks the liquid forward, down the tube and into the vessel. The rate of flow depends on the rotation speed of the rotor. When this factor remains constant, the precision of the device will be very good. Accuracy tends to be dependent on differences in lumen internal diameter among several tubes used from day to day. Changes in rate are made easily. The range of infusion rates covered by these changes also can be varied (Figure 15.4).

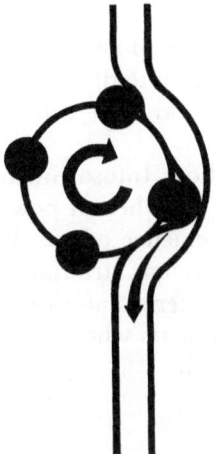

Figure 15.4 Each roller compresses the tubing so that it is closed, making an occlusive pump

The size and weight of this pump make it ideal for ambulatory infusion. It fits in the back pocket of gentleman's trousers or in the side pocket of a lady's blazer or in a pouch with a shoulder strap. The size of tubing which leads to the catheter is unobtrusive. Changes in the fluid reservoir (a small bag which is placed in the pump case) are made at 24–48 hour intervals, depending on the rate of flow selected from among several which are available. Adaptation of the patient to this device has been amazingly good. Each person seems to discover special tricks to handle the problems of fitting the infusion into their daily life style. Where several patients attend the same clinic, they trade stories and techniques, the 'old timer' always helping a recent initiate. These patients have a nearly normal life style, and when their disease responds to the treatment, the total result is truly gratifying.

An innovation has appeared recently which adds another dimension to ambulatory intravascular infusion. Called the Travenol 24 hour Infusor™ (Figure 15.3), it consists of a balloon which can be filled with fluid that is expressed through a fixed orifice. The key to its successful operation was the discovery of how to make these oblong balloons so that a constant pressure was exerted on the fluid as the quantity remaining diminished during the infusion period. Another critical feature was devising a method for mass production of the balloons in which each unit was a nearly exact copy of all others.

The Infusor is delivered from the manufacturer in an empty state. It is filled in the pharmacy with the medication to be given; 5% dextrose is added when necessary to make up a quantity of about 60 ml. Flow of liquid begins when the cap is removed from the integral administration set. It continues at a constant rate until all but 10 ml of liquid has been exhausted. At that point a diminished flow occurs until all the medication has run out. There is no rate modulation device on this unit. The first units have been set at the factory to deliver approximately 2 ml per hour (48 ml/day). However, size and flow rate variety likely will become available in the future.

The advantages of the 24 hour Infusor include (1) simplicity of operation, (2) total disposability, (3) inherent power source, (4) light weight, (5) small size, and (6) convenience of use. Pressures developed by the balloon are sufficient to overcome arterial pressure. There is a small decrease in flow when intra-arterial infusion is being made compared to intravenous delivery. The patients who have used this device have been uniformly enthusiastic about it.

CONTINUOUS INTRAVENOUS INFUSION (AMBULATORY)

The technique for accomplishing continuous ambulatory intravenous infusion combines components from routine intravenous infusions and the intra-arterial modality already discussed. There are two critical components, maintenance of a safe and patent vascular access for many days and provision of a delivery method that allows the patient full freedom of movement and a reasonably normal life style.

Stiff catheters are not used for intravenous infusions because there is no need to manipulate or direct the tip. In Chapter 9, Catheters, mention was made of silicone devices. These catheters exemplify the ultimate in their value when used for continuous intravenous infusion. Because the silicone elastomer induces almost no tissue reaction, it can remain in place for days or months as long as it is given reasonable care. For intravenous infusions the Intrasil product provides access to the vein at the antecubital fossa and a termination in the superior vena cava. Physicians at the M. D. Anderson Hospital have reported many patients with successful Intrasil dwell times measured in months and even years. The pliable and supple quality of the silicone produces no enduring discomfort for the patient. The Hickman catheter, placed in the subclavian position, also works very well for long term infusion, and my colleagues and I have had experience with several hundred patients using this device.

Pumps of the type described for intra-arterial therapy are suited equally to continuous intravenous infusion. Both the small battery powered MVP unit and the 'shrinking balloon' 24 hour Infusor give satisfactory results. Volumes usually administered are in the range of 25–50 ml daily. Drug reservoirs are changed at least every 48 hours.

Recently, we have reported on a series of patients with colo–rectal cancer who had metastasis to other vital organs (liver, lung) and areas (retroperitoneum, pelvis). These individuals were treated with the antitumor chemical 5-fluorouracil (5FU) administered by a continuous infusion for 20–540 days. The overall rate of tumor response was 40% (20% additional patients had stabile disease) which compares favorably with the usual response to 5FU given intermittently (15–20%). There were substantially fewer treatment side-effects. Other investigators have reported that vinca alkaloids, (a class of antitumor chemicals) and bleomycin and adriamycin (antitumor antibiotics) are given advantageously by continuous intravenous infusion.

One theory which is used to justify continuous infusion is that by maintaining a constant blood level of the chemical the malignant cells are exposed at a time when they are most susceptible to destruction. Another reason is that continuous infusion maintains a level for drugs which normally disappear rapidly from the bloodstream (have a short half life). A final thought has been that toxicity produced by some drugs may be caused by peak levels resulting from rapid or short term infusions. When a constant infusion is used, there are no high peaks of concentration.

I believe there is merit to each of these hypotheses. In many instances more than one might be operative. More research will be necessary, but it seems certain that continuous ambulatory intravenous infusion has found a place in intravascular infusion systems.

Some patients have been equipped with a system to administer 3000 ml of parenteral nutrition fluid per day while they are not in the hospital and remain ambulatory. This technique requires approximately 1000 ml of fluid to be carried on the body, usually in pockets of a vest-like garment. While it can be said this approach fits the concept of continuous ambulatory intravenous infusion, seeing such a patient caused me to appreciate the extent to which an individual will go to discard the fetters of a hospital environment. Such are the burdens of illness.

The primary complications of continuous intravenous infusion are vascular and infectious. Thrombosis of a vein or embolus have caused difficulties in a few patients. However, the most common adversity is systemic infection. It does not occur frequently. We have managed a series of over 100 patients with only one infection. For some unexplained reason, infection complications are not as frequent as among patients receiving parenteral nutrition.

As more physicians learn to manage these systems for the benefit of their patients, a steady increase in use will occur. The primary goal will be to shorten an expensive hospital stay. Another purpose will be to give medication in an optimal way.

179

CONTINUOUS SUBCUTANEOUS INSULIN INFUSION

This section is the only departure from subject matter described by the title of this book. However, the promise of continuous infusion of insulin for improved management of the diabetic justifies its inclusion as a new and exciting technology. In addition, much of the equipment being used is adapted from intravascular infusions.

After Banting and Best first described, isolated, and administered insulin to a diabetic dog, many thousands of diabetics were·granted a reprieve from early death due to the consequences of uncontrolled hyperglycemia. As clinical experience accumulated, it has become apparent that more subtle complications of diabetes often shorten life expectancy. Several specialists in diabetes believe better control of blood glucose might result in the mitigation of complications such as retinopathy leading to blindness, neuropathy, and vasculitis. Studies reported recently seem to demonstrate continuous subcutaneous infusion of regular insulin can produce a daily blood glucose curve in the diabetic which is quite similar to the non-diabetic patient. There is some expectation and a modicum of accumulated evidence that truly normalizing blood glucose improves at least early tissue changes of diabetes in the kidney and eye.

The method of infusion is simple. A small size needle (25 or 27 g) is inserted into the subcutaneous tissue of the abdomen and fastened in place with tape. A plastic connecting tube extends from the needle hub to a pump which the patient carries in a pocket or attaches to a belt. The pump has a reservoir for fluid, often a syringe which has been filled with regular insulin having a concentration that works compatibly with available pump speeds. The infusion rate is 1–2 ml for 24 hours. Supplementary bolus doses of insulin are self-administered at or very near meal times to counteract the sugar absorbed from food. These intermittent doses are given by increasing the pump speed for several minutes and then restoring the basal flow.

The proliferation of continuous insulin infusion has been remarkable, given the evidence available for its efficacy. The field of diabetes has waited a long time for a 'breakthrough' which could establish a new plateau of patient benefit; it may be that one has emerged.

CONTROLLED INTERMITTENT INFUSION

The need for well controlled intermittent infusion of several drugs has become apparent recently. It is known some drugs can be used more safely (such as gentamicin and tobramycin) when they are administered in this manner. The frequency of dosing may be two to six times daily. If left to manual control, it is easy to conceive how there may be substantial variability in timing and duration of doses. Automation is the key technique to manage this problem, which when handled well is an opportunity for improved patient care. Coming onto the market now are some pumps which can be programmed for duration, volume and frequency of infusion. These devices will maximize the potential for good parenteral drug control and minimize dosage errors. They will save valuable nurse and clinical pharmacist time, and will permit adaptation of emerging pharmacokinetics programs to patient care.

Bibliography

1. Balla, G. A., Mallams, J. T., Hutton, S., Arnoff, B. L. and Byrd, L. (1962). The treatment of head and neck malignancies by continuous intra-infusion of methotrexate. *Am. J. Surg.*, **104,** 699
2. Ausman, R. K., Caballero, G. C., Quebbeman, E. J. and Ausman, D. C. (1982). Long term ambulatory continuous intravenous infusion of 5-fluorouracil for treatment of metastatic adenocarcinoma of the liver. *Wisconsin Med. J.*, **81,** 25
3. Tamborlane, W. V., Sherwin, R. S., Korvisto, V. *et al.* (1979). Normalization of the growth hormone and catecholamine response to exercise in juvenile onset diabetic subjects treated with a portable insulin infusion pump. *Diabetes*, **28,** 785
4. Pickup, J. C. (1980). A new approach to improved metabolic control in diabetics: continuous subcutaneous insulin infusion. *Am. Heart J.*, **100,** 417

Appendix 1

SAMPLE PERIPHERAL CATHETER INSERTION AND CARE PROTOCOL

(1) Wash your hands with soap and water at the beginning of the procedure.

(2) Use an upper extremity for the insertion site.

(3) If hair removal is necessary, do not shave the area. Use scissors or a clipper.

(4) Scrub the proposed site with tincture of iodine, chlorhexidine, an iodophor or 70% alcohol. Allow the liquid to remain in contact with the skin for 30–60 seconds prior to vein puncture.

(5) Do not recontaminate the area by finger palpation.

(6) After the catheter is in place and flow into the vein is demonstrated, clean any blood from the skin surface and anchor the catheter in the prescribed manner. Do not put tape near the skin puncture, and do not cover the course of the catheter in the vein with tape so that adequate palpation is impossible. A sterile gauze dressing should be applied. Total occlusion by mounds of tape and gauze is unnecessary and unwise.

(7) Write the date of insertion, catheter type and size on the tape. Make the same record in the medical chart. Schedule the catheter for change.

(8) Examine the area of insertion at the same time each day, and write the date and time on the tape and in the medical chart to indicate the inspection has been performed. Check for early signs of phlebitis each time vital signs are observed.

(9) Change the catheter in 72 hours or less from the time of insertion. Immediately change catheters that have been placed in less than optimal circumstances.

(10) If the catheter is removed because of a concern for infection, it should be handled according to sterile technique rules so the *in vivo* portion can be cultured to determine the possible presence of contaminants. Routine removals need not be cultured.

SAMPLE PERIPHERAL CATHETER INSERTION AND CARE
PROTOCOL

Appendix 2

SUBCLAVIAN DRESSING CHANGE PROCEDURE

C. Teich, RN, MSN

GOALS OF THE DRESSING CHANGE PROCEDURE:

(1) To keep the catheter insertion site free of infection and dry.

(2) To handle new dressings so they will not be contaminated.

THE MAJOR STEPS OF THE DRESSING CHANGE PROCEDURE INCLUDE:

(1) Removing the old dressing and discarding it,

(2) Inspecting the insertion site,

(3) Cleansing the area, and

(4) Redressing the insertion site.

EQUIPMENT AND SUPPLIES:

(1) Hydrogen peroxide,

(2) Sterile cotton swabs (6–8),

(3) Iodine ointment (bacitracin can be used if allergic to iodine),

(4) Sterile 2″×2″ or 4″×4″ gauze pads, and

(5) Tape (or a plastic dressing).

PROCEDURE:

(1) Wash hands well.

(2) Remove old dressing and inspect area for
   – redness
   – swelling
   – drainage
   – tenderness

(3) Clean insertion site of catheter with hydrogen peroxide using circular motions moving from insertion site outwards to an area of approximately 3–4″ wide.

(4) Apply ointment with a cotton-tipped applicator to the insertion site. (optional).

(5) Apply a new dressing. Often a single sheet transparent dressing is sufficient.

(6) Tape—use the type best suited for the patient. Use a plastic dressing if desired.

(7) Change dressing every other day or 3 times weekly if gauze dressing is used, and once a week if a plastic dressing is used. If area becomes wet, change the dressing.

Reference

Hickman, R. O. and Bjeletich, J. (1980). The Hickman Indwelling Catheter. *Am. J. Nursing*, Jan: 62

Appendix 3

ON THE ROLE OF STATISTICAL SAMPLING IN ADMIXTURE QUALITY ASSURANCE PROGRAMS

R. L. Sanford, Ph.D.

End-product testing for microbial contamination as part of quality assurance programs for admixture services has been discussed by the National Coordinating Committee on Large Volume Parenterals. Bacterial surveillance and sterility monitoring have been discussed by Buth and Ravin. Since only 100% error-free, non-destructive inspection and testing of admixtures would ensure that no defective, non-sterile product leaves an admixture service, end-product testing can only serve as part of a quality assurance program safeguarding the patient. Depending on the objectives to be served, different inspection and testing regimes can be devised. Statistical sampling plans can provide feedback on the frequency of occurrence of positive sterility tests so that unacceptable shifts in the non-sterility rate can be detected with known statistical risks. The role of such procedures in admixture quality assurance programs needs comment.

STATISTICAL AIDS TO SUPPORT QUALITY ASSURANCE

Control of quality results from the detection and elimination of factors which cause product defects. Deming has pointed out that causes of unacceptable product can be subsumed under two categories:

(1) Faults of the system (which are common to more than one worker or machine),

(2) Special causes (which are specific to a certain worker or to a machine).

Deming has indicated faults of the system, in his experience, overshadow special causes in importance. Both categories require the attention of management.

Statistical methods can aid management in detecting causes of unacceptable products relative to a standard. Statistical methods aid in placing the responsibility where it belongs, problem by problem, be that with the system or some special cause. In those cases where the workers are handicapped by the system and predisposed to making a defective product, only a change in the system can effect a solution. Other causes may be correctable by the workers. Phrasing it differently, establishing a standard of admixture quality involves designing a system which is capable of producing an acceptable product. Maintaining this quality level involves controlling the system to insure reliable operation. Statistical methods can be used to detect significant departures from the norm. These departures may result from the system or have special origins. If the system is the probable cause, control or improvement in admixture quality involves devising better methods of production. If the probable cause has a special origin such as a particular worker, attention to the specific individual is required. This leads to a very important process of administration.

SYSTEMS ANALYSIS — HOW TO GET STARTED

For statistical methods to aid management, a structure must be developed that finds relevant problems. It is fundamental to begin by studying the system of admixture preparation. Different modes of preparation should be identified which differ, for example, in terms of steps, techniques, people and equipment employed. Product types should be classified by mode of preparation. Each product category resulting from a particular mode of preparation is potentially subject to monitoring. The rationale for this approach is that it serves to partially sort out the set of causes (system and special) that pertain to one product category relative to other product categories. Pragmatic judgment must be used in specifying these categories. This discussion will assume each product unit in a given category to have the same probability of contamination. By statistically sampling each production stream so identified and using statistical algorithms to determine if the non-sterility rate has shifted, corrective action can be initiated when it is needed and focused at the set of potential causes associated with the product category involved.

MONITORING PRODUCTION STREAMS

Recommendations regarding a particular type of sampling plan well adapted to the needs of admixture quality control have been given elsewhere. This type of sampling plan is called a Cumulative Sum (CuSum) control chart, and allows charting of non-sterility test results. If the quality level is measured as a non-sterility rate, this approach allows discrimination between an acceptable quality level and a rejectable quality level with a specified statistical error rate. Cumulative Sum (CuSum) charts are more effective than comparable Shewhart charts in picking up a sudden persistent change of moderate magnitude in the process non-sterility rate. Cumulative Sum (CuSum) charts are not appropriate for analyzing data exhibiting cyclic variation.

Since the specifics of constructing a CuSum chart have been given

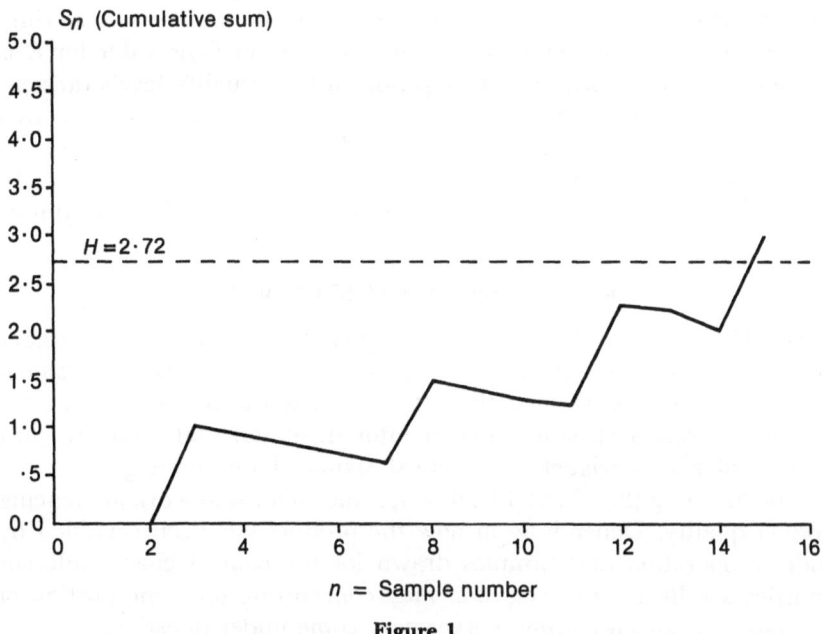

Figure 1

elsewhere, only the briefest overview will be offered here. Figure 1 illustrates such a chart. For admixture sterility testing results, imagine product units being sampled at random from the finished product stream over a period of time. A statistic S_n is computed.

$$S_n = \sum_{i=1}^{n} (X_i - K)$$

where,

S_n = cumulative sum

n = number of units sampled and tested

$X_i = \begin{cases} 0 \text{ if } i^{th} \text{ units sterile} \\ 1 \text{ if } i^{th} \text{ unit non-sterile} \end{cases}$

K = reference level.

If S_n ever equals zero or goes negative, it is set to zero and the computation process restarted with the next sample test result. The n test results accumulated to this point are forgotten. The value of S_n is compared against a constant H called the decision point or boundary. If S_n exceeds H, an out-of-control situation has been detected. The value for K is determined by formulae to reflect the acceptable and rejectable quality levels for the process in question. For sterility monitoring, the acceptable quality level might be the non-sterility false positive rate for

189

the test used. The rejectable quality level is some greater non-sterility rate which must be detected quickly if it does occur. The value for H is also determined by formulae. H depends on both quality levels (acceptable and rejectable), as well as on the frequency of false alarms generated by random chance which will be tolerated. The larger the value for H, the less frequent a false alarm will be generated by random chance. In Figure 1, an out-of-control state was detected with the fifteenth sample.

MANAGEMENT IMPLICATIONS

When a CuSum control chart (or some other statistical aid) is used under the circumstances described, management will receive a statistical signal that a shift has occurred in the rate of non-sterile test results for the particular product stream being monitored. Solitary false positive test results will rarely trigger a statistical signal. Thus, management can respond knowing that, in all likelihood, some factor is at work influencing product quality. Depending on how the product has been classified by mode of operation and samples drawn for the control chart, different inquiries are likely. Investigation may concentrate on some portion of the system or an individual worker may come under question.

It is common industrial practice to focus on individual workers, bringing to their attention each defective product. Such a practice is not encouraged by this writer. The important point made earlier was that only statistically significant changes in quality should be studied. If a technician is in a state of statistical control holding his performance level constant, using a CuSum chart to monitor his performance should lead to infrequent false signals that a change has occurred. For such workers, Deming has indicated that further education or practice in technique will not lead to much improvement in performance. Such workers have established their level of skill. Education or practice in technique may help people who are not in control establish a stable level of performance. If this does not happen, management may need to assign people to other jobs if they cannot achieve a suitable state of control and level of performance in order to maintain quality. This philosophy pertains to the practice of forcing requalification of aseptic technique by the worker involved whenever a sterility test positive turns up for one of his product units. Such a practice may not be that helpful. If a technician has naturally good technique, he will, in all probability, pass a requalification without improvement in technique. If a technician has a higher than average non-sterility rate but is in statistical control, forcing requalification is unlikely to help lower his average non-sterility rate. Rather than spend money for requalifications, reassignment of the person makes more sense. The technician who is still improving his technique may benefit by achieving greater control over his work. In each case, a statistical signal should be used to determine when management needs to intervene to correct a change in performance. The technician with sound technique will rarely be bothered. Others will be flagged more frequently. Responsibility will be placed where it should be.

CONCLUSION

Use of a sampling inspection plan is meant to ensure that product quality will meet a pre-established standard. Inspection should serve two purposes, according to Dodge:

(1) It provides a basis for direct action on existing product, and
(2) It provides a basis for action on the production process to maintain or improve quality in the future.

Provided sampling results are evaluated with statistical methods to produce sound decisions for action, efforts can be directed toward identifying and correcting faults in the admixture production process. Such faults may be in the system or of some special origin. The result of such an unrelenting effort to correct the causes of defects will be improved product quality.

References

1. National Coordinating Committee on Large Volume Parenterals. (1980). Recommended guidelines for quality assurance in hospital centralized intravenous admixture services. *Am. J. Hosp. Pharm.*, **37,** 645
2. Buth, J. A., Coberly, R. W. and Eckel, F. M. (1973). A practical method of sterility monitoring of IV admixtures and a method of implementing a routine sterility monitoring program. *Drug Intell. Clin. Pharm.*, **17,** 276
3. Ravin, R., Bahr, J., Luscomb, F. *et al.* (1974). Program for bacterial surveillance of intravenous admixtures. *Am. J. Hosp. Pharm.*, **31,** 340
4. Deming, W. E. (1975). On some statistical aids toward economic production. *Interfaces*, **5,** No. 4
5. Sanford, R. L. (1980). Cumulative sum control charts for admixture quality control. *Am. J. Hosp. Pharm.*, **37,** 655
6. Van Dobben De Bruyn, C. S. (1968). *Cumulative sum tests.* (New York: Hafner Publishing)
7. Woodward, R. H. and Goldsmith, P. L. (1964). *Cumulative Sum Techniques.* (Edinburgh: Oliver and Boyd)
8. Dodge, H. F. (1950). Inspection for quality assurance. *Ind. Qual. Control*, **7,** 6

Index